FAT, SICK & NEARLY DEAD

# FAT, SICK & NEARLY DEAD

## HOW FRUITS & VEGETABLES
## CHANGED MY LIFE

## BY JOE CROSS

Foreword by Joel Fuhrman, M.D. & Afterword by Dean Ornish, M.D.

All Still photos (except from Joe's personal collection):
Daniel Marracino.

Screen grabs taken from the movie "Fat, Sick
& Nearly Dead"

Animations: FlickerLab for Fat, Sick & Nearly Dead

ISBN
978-1-4507-6478-0
978-1-4507-6479-7

TO ALL THOSE PEOPLE
BRAVE ENOUGH TO TRY

# ACKNOWLEDGMENTS

I want to thank all those who worked with me on the book, as well as all those I met along the way, including Phil Staples, his brother Barry "Bear" Staples, and Bear's wife, Claudia. I couldn't have accomplished any of this without them, or without my family and friends.

Leigh Haber helped me conceive, write, and edit the book. I am very grateful to her for her partnership, dedication, and superb editorial skills. It's a book!

To Stacey Offman, Jamin Mendelsohn, and Jessica Mennella—the heart and soul of the Reboot team—my deep thanks.

Naomi Mizusaki expertly art directed the book and Helena Holgersson-Shorter lent her extraordinary copyediting skills. Chika Azuma was a lifesaver. Thanks to them, as well as to the team at Blurb.

Stacy Kennedy, senior clinical nutritionist at the Brigham & Young Women's Hospital/Dana Farber Cancer Institute; superstar authors Joel Fuhrman, M.D. and Dean Ornish, M.D., and my brother, Tom Cross, M.D. all provided invaluable contributions and are an inspiration.

I also owe a debt of gratitude to Andrew Rasiej, Alison Riley, Professor Ronald Penny, Amie Hannon, Chris Seward, John Alexander, Scott Willett, Susan Ainsworth, Lisa McLean, Stephanie Atkinson, Cameron Paine-Thaler, Shane Hodson, Vicky Elkins, Millie Katter, Kurt Engfehr, Daniel Marracino, Christopher Seward, Norma Kamali, Robert Mac, Nicola Simmonds, K.Emily Bond, Irene Deutsch, Charles and Belinda Dowsett, John Cross, and my parents Merv and Virginia Cross, who have set the example and leadership that I try to aspire to every day of my life.

# TABLE OF CONTENTS

# FOREWORD BY
# DR. JOEL FUHRMAN

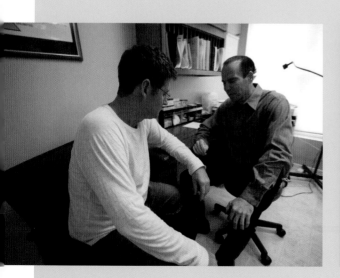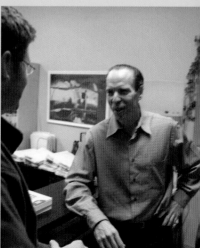

Americans have become among the sickliest, most overweight generation in the history of the human race. Our children's generation can expect a shocking increase in early life mortality. The primary reason? We Americans are eating our way into sickness and premature death, and many others throughout the world are following suit. Joe Cross is determined to help reverse this trend, as he did in his own life, via something as simple but essential as eating fruits and vegetables and minimizing his consumption of meat, caffeine, dairy, sugar, and processed foods..

Between 1935 and 2005, for seventy years straight, the occurrence of cancers that can be definitively linked to obesity—cancers of the colon, breast, endometrial lining, and kidneys, for example—have increased every year. When you stop to think about this, this is a near incomprehensible statistic, which, I believe, can be traced directly to the creation of junk, processed, and fast "foods," foods we have become addicted to. It is not a coincidence that at the same time, the incidence of autoimmune diseases is skyrocketing and we are witnessing an epidemic of chronic diseases of what I call "nutritional ignorance." In fact, nutrition-related deaths among the overweight malnourished are becoming as prevalent as deaths among those in the world who don't get enough to eat. And it is very often the malnourished overweight— those who are taking in huge amounts of calories but still not getting the nutrition their bodies need to thrive and ward off disease—who eventually find their way to the doors of my medical practice.

By the time many of my patients arrive at my office they are already in the midst of full-blown medical crises. Why? The statistics tell the story: the average American woman today, for example, weighs a full forty pounds more than her counterpart one hundred years ago and has a vastly higher rate of heart attack, stroke, and breast cancer. Among American men, the incidence of death by cardiac arrest has quadrupled over the same period. American men today are ten times more likely to have a heart attack. Overall, more than a third of the American population will die of a heart attack or stroke, which make those the leading cause of death in the U.S. Just one hundred years ago, this figure was below five percent.

Let's look at this from a nutritional standpoint, as what we are eating (and what we aren't eating) is directly causing the illnesses that are killing us. Our diets have become centered on the consumption of cheese, pasta, meat, bread, fried foods, and sugar-filled snacks and drinks. The potato is the most commonly eaten vegetable, usually in the form of chips or French fries. Many of these foods have been "processed," which among other things means they are high in calories and low in nutritive value. Meanwhile, we are consuming very little in the way of plant-based, micronutrient-rich foods, which have the power to promote health and prevent disease. USDA food consumption data indicate that unrefined plant foods comprise less than ten percent of our total caloric intake. Processed and fast foods, sweets and oils are rich in calories, yet low in disease-protecting micronutrients, but it is these foods that have become our mainstays. Our addictions to these "foods" are holding us hostage and directly creating the immense suffering and medical tragedies I see in my patients, fueling a medical crisis that cannot be solved simply by the addition of more and more prescription drugs. We are digging our own graves using our knives and forks.

Our poor nutritional habits have an effect not only on our physical health, but on our larger society. The burden of massive medical costs for treating conditions produced by our poor health is weighing down our economy and even helping to drive jobs overseas. What's more, studies show that more than twenty-five percent of defaults on mortgages and home rentals are actually a result of medical debt. So what's to be done?

In the face of this all-out American health crisis—a crisis that is quickly spreading around the world—our government and medical leaders are offering us more access to medical care and medications. Are drugs really the solution to the explosion of obesity, diabetes, heart disease, and cancer we are experiencing? Or is it the cause of these problems—a disease-creating lifestyle and diet—that we should be taking a much harder look at? The real foundation of healthcare—healthcare that gives individuals control of their health destinies and is truly effective in restoring good health, without heart disease, diabetes and cancer– must be proper nutrition and a high quality food supply.

What if I told you that it is possible to prevent more than 95% of all deaths from cardiovascular disease and 80% of all cancer deaths simply via excellent nutrition? 1.1 million Americans will suffer heart attacks this year, tragedies that are completely unnecessary. Nobody HAS to die of heart disease or of a circulatory system-related death. Such deaths are nearly always preventable. The disability, suffering, and life years lost as a result of these conditions are almost entirely the product of dietary/ nutritional ignorance. Making a transition to healthy eating can literally reverse the progress of some chronic diseases; can prevent heart disease, diabetes, stroke, and even cancer; can dramatically extend lifespan and healthy life expectancy. Nutritional excellence can enable people to stop being dependent on medications and help them to make profound, dramatic recoveries, even from serious illnesses such as asthma, chronic migraines, lupus, fibromyalgia, and arthritis. Nutritional science has advanced to the point where this goal is in sight.

We must start towards this goal one person at a time, which is one of the reasons I applaud and support what Joe Cross is doing. He began with the goal of saving his own life, and now hopes to turn what he's learned into a movement. But it hasn't always been easy for him, nor is it for my other patients. Time and time again, I have encountered patients who have all but given up, who believe that their days of good health and vitality are behind them. They have grown tired of trying to lose weight, feel beaten down by the side effects of their prescription drugs, which they have to take every day just to keep going. They may remember what it was like to feel energetic and full of life, but have begun to settle for mere survival. Watching these people transform themselves by harnessing the innate healing properties of the human body, as Joe Cross did via his self-styled Reboot, has been tremendously exciting and rewarding. You, too, can achieve a state of optimal health, but like Joe, you'll have to earn it. The message of this book and of Joe's related movie, *Fat, Sick & Nearly Dead*, is that our bodies are miraculous, self-healing machines that when properly fed and cared for can enable us to take back control of our health and get well. We can become the healthiest people on the planet instead of being among the sickest and fattest.

When I first met Joe Cross, he was another of the many long-suffering victims of chronic illness I meet every day in my practice. He was not just overweight, he also had a painful autoimmune disease. Through research and trial and error, he had learned a lot about the essential value of a plant-based diet and of the destructive power of many of the fake "foods" that have been developed over the last one hundred years. However, he had not yet been able to consistently integrate this knowledge into his daily life, though he was trying. Joe is Australian, (Australians are giving Americans a run for their money in the quest to become the fattest people on the planet), a once-athletic guy who had shot past 300 pounds by age forty. Joe had also developed chronic urticaria—a painful autoimmune disease closely related to lupus, which increases one's risk of cancer later in life. His symptoms were being managed by taking a steroid called Prednisone which has many side effects, including weight gain, depression, and stomach ulcers. Joe was successful in virtually every area of his life except in the area of physical health. When I met him, he was tired of living with the effects of the disease and the Prednisone, and worried about his future quality of life. However, Joe is a very determined guy, and he had decided he had to make a radical and permanent change in order to heal himself. That's how he came up with the idea of the Reboot.

In many areas, moderation is a good thing. However, when it comes to how much of our diets should be made up of processed foods, junk food, and fast foods, I take a more extreme view: I believe that these things should be removed from our diets entirely. I do not approve of moderation in cancer-causing habits such as smoking or eating cancer-causing foods. As Joe's diet at the time contained a very high percentage of these non-food foods, eliminating them from his life would involve drastic action. Joe had decided he would kick things off by going on a sixty-day juice fast designed to "reboot" his system, giving him a chance to get off the harmful drugs he was taking as quickly as possible and helping him cultivate a new hunger for healthful, natural, real food. Sure, he chose a radical way to start, but a radical plan was something Joe needed to begin to make dramatic, permanent changes.

It has now been a few years since I first met Joe, and in the interim he has completely turned his health around. He has also written this book and produced a movie about the Reboot process and his journey back to health. Both projects are truly inspiring. These days Joe and I share a mission, which is to help people improve their health by enabling and encouraging those who desire freedom from the painful, disruptive, even fatal effects of nutritional ignorance to overcome their food addictions and their dependence on prescription drugs, so they can lead more comfortable, more pleasurable, longer lives.

Join us on our journey, or as Joe would say, "Juice on."

**Joel Fuhrman, M.D. is a renowned speaker and author of numerous bestselling books, including the influential *Eat to Live: The Revolutionary Plan for Fast and Sustained Weight Loss*. He is a board-certified family physician who specializes in preventing and reversing disease through nutritional and natural methods.**

# INTRODUCTION

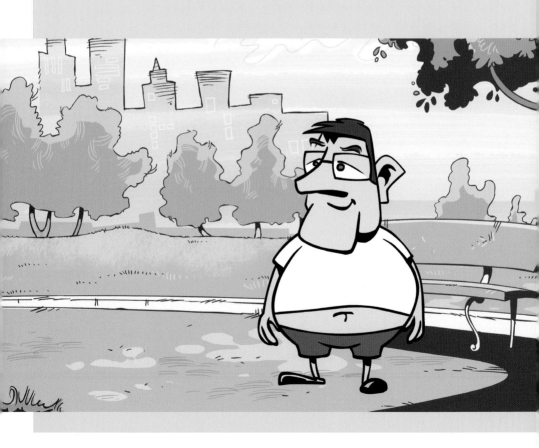

It is my view that in life, people are equipped with certain tools they can use to carve out their own paths. We go about our daily lives trying to use those tools as efficiently and as creatively as we can, muddling our way through the obstacles that conspire to prevent us from moving forward. At times we make good progress, at other times we make very little headway, or get stuck. There are moments when we can see the way ahead with great clarity, then inevitably, our paths once again get a little rockier and tougher to navigate. Sometimes when we lose sight of our goals we can fall back on our instincts to get us back on track, or the wisdom or experience of others to help us figure out which way to turn. But what if nothing seems to work? What if the tools we've always counted on to get us through life just stop working? It is at those times that we have to step back and take stock to try and get a sense of the bigger picture. If we were lost in a forest, we would perhaps find a tall tree and climb to the top in order to get some perspective—even to see whether or not we are in the right forest anymore!

Me, Joe Cross, at my heaviest, depicted in an animation from my film *FAT, SICK & NEARLY DEAD*

During paralyzing moments of confusion, when we are looking around, trying to regain our clarity and decide "what's next?"—it is at those crossroads when big decisions often get made and we find ourselves making promises to ourselves or others. While our intentions may be good, it is especially hard to move to the next stage of putting those promises and plans into action. That's how I felt for the longest time before I got started on this journey. I had the best intentions, but somehow I couldn't get from knowing what I needed to do to doing it.

I have a theory, which is that most of us spend the first forty years of our lives killing ourselves and the next forty trying to stay alive. If this an anthem of modern life then consider me the poster boy for that choir, because at the advanced age of forty-one I woke up to find myself *fat, sick, and nearly dead.* And when I say that, I am not being melodramatic.

Up until a couple of years ago, I was about as unhealthy as a forty-year-old can get. I was massively overweight, with an excruciatingly painful autoimmune disease called urticaria. Touch me and I puffed up. On a particularly bad day I could give the Elephant Man a run for his money, that's how bad it was. Between my weight and the urticaria, it had

Me during an uticaria outbreak, as depicted via animation in the film.

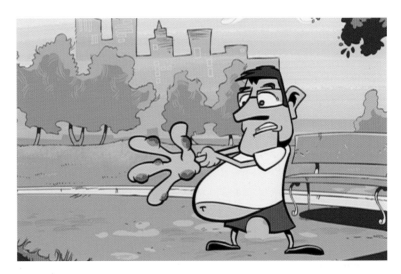

become just about impossible for me to do many of the things I most enjoyed in life. I couldn't play golf with my dad, I couldn't pick up my nieces and nephews in my arms to give them a hug, I couldn't have sex without causing an outbreak.

When I was first diagnosed in 1999, my doctors were concerned that if my windpipe should swell up from an outbreak, I could end up choking to death. Even the slightest pressure from a snug- fitting, starched shirt collar could actually be life-threatening. Not exactly the sort of heroic death one would choose for one's self. No one knew what was causing the urticaria, but there was a "miracle" drug I was prescribed for it none-theless. At the time, I didn't dwell on how illogical it was that there could be a drug prescribed for something the doctors couldn't figure out the cause of. Instead, I thought: "Well, hooray for miracle drugs, then!" Mine was called Prednisone, which is a very powerful immunosuppressant that can buy you some time when you need it. I had about ten years before the drug would officially begin to create more problems than it solved. Here are a few well-documented side effects of Prednisone: weight gain, osteoporosis, glaucoma, hepatic necrosis, Cushing's syn-drome (which causes "moon face"), cardiovascular enlargement, mania, black stools...you get the picture.

What soon became clear to me about Prednisone is that it's like using your credit card to get well. You're getting what looks like good health: for example, it stopped the Elephant Man from turning up to important business meetings or big dates on my behalf. But because this faux health is bought on credit, it has to be paid back with interest. Doctors don't recommend long-term use of Prednisone for some of the reasons noted above. And while I was grateful to have something that helped minimize the effects of the urticaria for nearly a decade, I never stopped feeling like a 300-pound "bubble boy" on steroids, desperately searching for a cure.

There are about as many opportunities out there to screw up your health as there are possible "cures." I've tried almost every one. Pretty much from the word "go" I've been a huge eater without a stop button, whether I was consuming more bottles of formula than my brothers and sister when we were babies, or devouring ice cream after ice cream, pizza after pizza, and Big Mac after Big Mac when I got older. I drank oceans of Coke and got very good at binge-drinking alcohol. As a matter of fact, there weren't a lot of mind-altering substances I said no to. You can bet I was always the first bloke at the table and the last to leave, and boy, did I pay the price. Every now and then I thought about making a change and so suddenly switched gears, searching high and low for ways to lose weight and get healthy. On the alternative side, I trawled through the A-Z of what the New Age healers had to offer, from acupuncture to hypnosis. I even went to a so-called voodoo doctor for his opinion. On the more traditional side, I tried diets, fasts, and of course, consulted with the best medical brain-power money could buy. I saw the top skin and autoimmune doctors in the world, but got no closer to a cure. They really didn't understand what was happening to me and kept using the same word to describe it. My disease was "idiopathic" in origin: in other words, no one knew where it came from or how to get rid of it.

To complete the mystery thriller atmosphere surrounding my poor health, I should tell you that I come from a family of medical professionals. My dad, Merv Cross, is one of Australia's leading knee surgeons; my brother, Tom, is a sports doctor who has worked with Olympians at the

**WHAT IS URTICARIA?** The type I have is a chronic autoimmune condition of unknown origin causing frequent outbreaks of painful, red hives. Ouch!

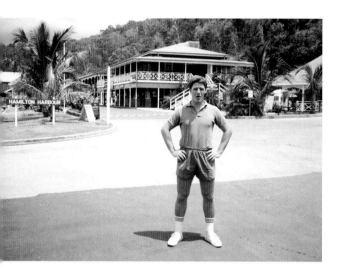 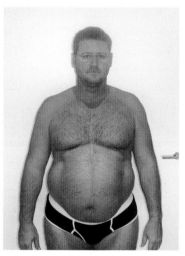

Me, in my early, fit, finest days, before things started going off the rails.

Me, off the rails

Institute of Sport in Canberra; my mother, Virginia, is a former nurse. Yet even they couldn't help me. This frustrated them, and especially tore my mother's heart out. I began to realize that I would have to try and take back control of my health—I couldn't leave it to Prednisone, to world-renowned specialists, or to my parents. The only question was, how?

I have always thought of a successful life as having five essential components: family and friends; work; love; self/spirituality; health. My view is that even if you are hugely successful in a couple of these catego-ries, but not very good in the others, then your life is out of balance. As I took stock of my own life at age forty and of how I'd gotten to this low point in terms of my health, I reflected that I had done pretty well in terms of that first category, friends and family. On a scale of one to ten, I could give myself a ten. Next came work. I had achieved success financially and professionally, more than I'd ever dreamed possible. I also assigned myself a ten in that area. The third area was a bit tougher to evaluate. I had had plenty of wonderful relationships, but not one that had lasted over the long term. To be honest, I had to give myself a five there. Similarly, when it came to self/spirituality, because I had devoted so much time to business over just about everything else, that was also no more than a five out of ten. As for my health—that was my true Achilles heel. I could only give myself a one out of ten points. Through my terrible eating habits (and the effects of the Prednisone) I had gradually gained weight throughout my twenties and thirties, complete with accompanying huge belly and triple chins. My binge drinking wasn't helping things either. In addition to the extra calories and the comfort food I ate to fight off the next morning's hangovers, when I drank, I got pretty obnoxious. I was one of those guys with a lot of cash in his pocket who tries to put every second girl in the bar into a headlock. To put it mildly, no one would have mistaken me for George Clooney during this period.

As I looked at my score of one in the health category, I wondered if the very fact that I was a ten in the work area was skewing the balance of everything else. Let's face it: when you are depressed or compulsive in certain behaviors, it is easy to hide behind work and convince yourself that as long as that's going well, nothing's really wrong. And that brings me to my decision to try and cure myself by going on an extended, detoxifying, cleansing juice fast, which I dubbed a "Reboot." This decision was born out of desperation and preparation: I had tried everything else and none of it had worked, but along the way, I'd begun to observe some patterns that led me to believe that somehow fruits and vegetables would be my partners in the journey to wellness.

That's how I found myself in the United States, spending two months exploring the country with film crew and juicer in tow, making an autobiographical film about a sixty-day, cross-country "Reboot." Nope, there's no punch line to that. The film is actually about me on a two-month-long juice fast. But you know something? It turned out pretty well. The film is called *Fat, Sick & Nearly Dead*, which as you know, describes my state before I decided to try and change my life and share the process with an audience by making a movie using money out of my own pocket. No matter how crazy it sounds, though, the plan worked. By going back to basics, by going back to the foods that come most directly from Mother Nature, I was able to reclaim the healthy Joe I'd almost lost for good and to retire my Prednisone. In the course of making the film, I traveled the back roads of the United States, meeting a lot of very nice people and other average Joes, who, like me, were just trying to get a grip on their health. I interviewed many of them for the film and I learned a lot along the way. I hope that by sharing my journey with them—and with you—I am offering firsthand proof that your good health is truly in your own hands. Can something as simple as getting back to eating foods that are good for you really cure you of something the best doctors in the world can't figure out how to fix? The answer is yes. The solution was right there in front of me all along. But sometimes, even when you know deep down that something is true, it doesn't sink in until you actually prove it to yourself.

By the way, the end of my sixty-day Reboot was really just the beginning. Once my physical body detoxed during the Reboot process, my mind became astonishingly clear. I began to plan how I would move forward from there. Would I be able to truly and permanently change the way I lived my life? The Reboot put that choice back in my hands. It returned me to the driver's seat, and that is what I hope it will do for you.

## SO, WHAT IS A REBOOT?

Reboot — A time to recharge and get your body and your diet back in alignment with nature. A period of time where you commit to eating and drinking only fruits, vegetables, and water in order to regain your vitality and kick-start healthy habits.

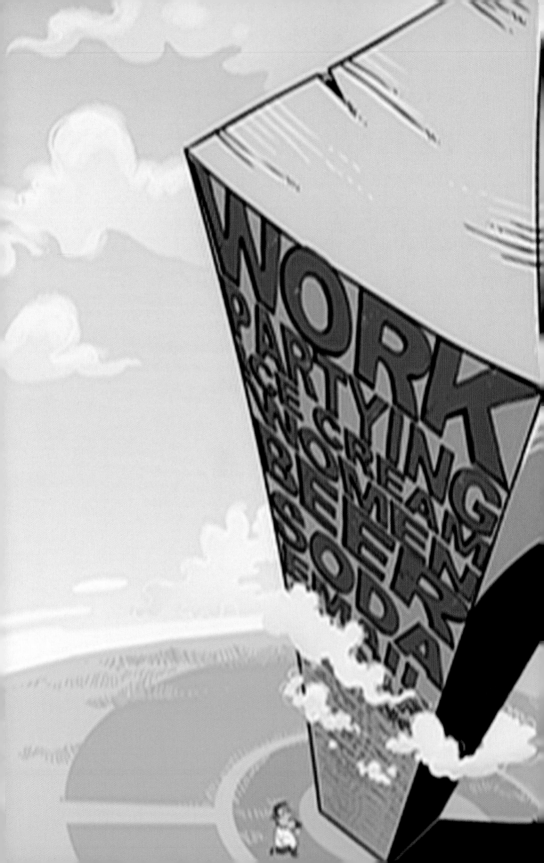

# CHAPTER ONE

# I CHOSE WEALTH OVER HEALTH

IN MY EARLY TWENTIES I WAS EARNING HUNDREDS OF THOUSANDS OF DOLLARS PER YEAR AND LIVING A BOOM-OR-BUST LIFE.

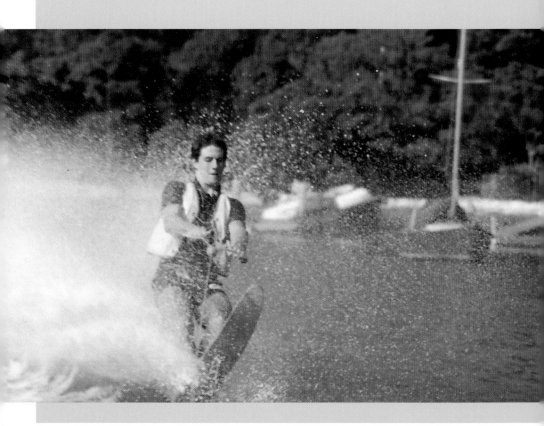

When I was growing up, I ate pretty much anything I wanted and most of what I wanted had sugar in it. Looking back, I'm pretty sure I was addicted to sugar; it really gave me a high. As a result, I don't have a single molar in my mouth that doesn't have a filling, or hasn't been replaced because it rotted out from the constant onslaught of sugar.

My brothers and sister and I pretty much ate whatever we wanted, and we did so with gusto at the same time burning off the calories with all our sporting activities.

Our family's eating habits were typical of an Australian family of that time: three meals a day, starting with breakfast, including lots of cereal, probably sugar-based. Most of our dinners included some form of meat along with at least three vegetables. Leg of lamb was on the menu once a week or more.

Mum didn't allow us to have sugar-based drinks such as Coca-Cola except for special treats. I looked forward to another weekly treat: after Mass Sunday evenings we went to to Mc Donalds, which is where I developed my love affair with the big Mac. And Mum changed her mind about Coca-Cola as I entered my teenage years, thinking if I got to drink Coke I might not turn to alcohol!

By the way, I don't fault my parents for this—they were just doing what parents do, which was to be sure we were well-fed and happy. I can remember as a kid feeling surprised—even shocked—whenever I went to a neighbor's house and saw a fully stocked supply of food when I opened the refrigerator. It wasn't that our mother never bought food, it was just that our constant refrigerator raids would clean out its contents within hours of a trip to the grocery store. It was hard for me to imagine being in a family that didn't eat as massively and voraciously as we did. Restraint and discipline were not in my vocabulary, at least not when it came to food. The closest I came to eating fruits and vegetables was the lettuce and onion on my Big Mac, something that, as it turns out, is pretty typical of many kids growing up.

My father worked long hours building his medical practice in Australia, while my mother stayed home raising us. Before we settled down, my family moved around a lot—we even spent a year living in Columbus,

Georgia, U.S.A.—while my father completed his medical residency in orthopedics. By the time I was in fifth grade I'd attended a total of five schools. Every move came with a huge adjustment and produced more than a little insecurity in me. I got into quite a few fights at school; I won more fights than I lost, but rarely felt like a winner. When I got home, though, I could always count on food to provide a healing tonic.

I can remember coming home from school and emptying an entire box of cereal into a mixing bowl, drowning it all in milk and heaping mounds of sugar on top. As we all know, when it comes to breakfast cereals, the cardboard box often contains more nutrition than the actual cereal: at least this was true for the brands I favored. I repeated this ritual on a daily basis, parking myself in front of the television, bowl in lap, to watch my favorite TV shows. My viewing schedule went something like this:

4:00 p.m.: *Gilligan's Island*
4:30 p.m.: *I Dream of Jeannie*
5:00 p.m.: *Hogan's Heroes*
5:30 p.m.: *The Brady Bunch*
6:00 p.m.: *Get Smart*
6:30 p.m.: *Bewitched*

That two-and-a-half hours before dinnertime was like a retreat to my own private resort, complete with an all-you-can-eat buffet.

As I grew older, burgers began to replace sugar as my first love. Even in my early teens I could manage to eat three entire burgers in a single sitting. My favorite combo was a Big Mac, two cheeseburgers, and an order of French fries washed down with a chocolate shake and a small Coke. I can still recall one occasion when, on a dare, I attempted to eat twenty Big Macs in a row. I only got to eleven, though I reckon if it hadn't been for the pickles I could have gone all the way. Fortunately, I was naturally very lean, athletic, and generally always on the move when I was in high school. My bad habits wouldn't start catching up with me until later.

When I was old enough to add alcohol to my daily diet, I pretty much spiraled out of control. I started gaining a lot of weight as I gradually

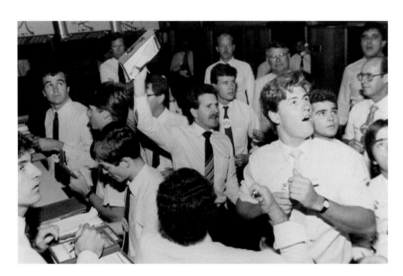

That's me on the floor of the Sydney Futures Exchange with other Masters of The Universe

traded in my good health and athletic physique for partying and physical suffering. In many ways, though, it was hard to complain because I considered myself to be very lucky in terms of what I was able to achieve at a very early age, namely, independent wealth.

I started playing the stock market and betting on horses when I was fourteen. I was very close to my grandfather, Don Cross, who schooled me in the principles of risk and reward using a betting form as a guide. For most Australians, horse racing and betting is in our DNA, and I spent a lot of my early adolescence on the phone with my grandfather, debating which horses to back. I usually spread out my money over eight races at fifty cents a bet, and listened to the races on the radio via an earpiece I hid from my teachers. Win or lose, the thrill of not getting caught was half the fun. My family was all about medicine and didn't care about the machinations of the stock market, but that didn't deter me. I spent a lot of time "pretending" to buy and sell stock by closely following certain companies in the newspaper.

What this love of gambling, risk, and reward confirmed in me was that I had a thing for numbers. It was the sort of gift that didn't require me to go to university to develop it, so after high school, at age eighteen, I applied for a job as a runner on the floor of the Sydney Futures Exchange.

# "Ah, the good old days!"

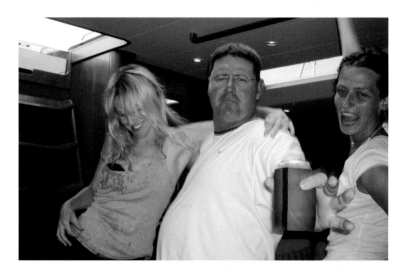

The advertised job promised a "life in the fast lane" for the successful applicant, who turned out to be me. I learned this game quickly, becoming, at nineteen, one of the youngest traders to receive a full trading license. While most of my mates were in college having parties, meeting girls, and opening their first bank accounts, I was being taught how to handle and manipulate millions of dollars of other people's money. It was a natural high very few teenagers get to experience. And by the way, it was the eighties, when greed ruled the game with Gordon Gekko as team captain.

Australians deviated from Wall Street customs in a few ways. For example, taking a lunch break was not scorned on the Australian Street. Rather, it was considered a ripe opportunity to drink three or four bottles of wine and then to work drunk for the rest of the afternoon. "Real men" came back to the office and handled it. Only wimps went home early to nurse their late-afternoon hangovers. To get that drunk and get away with it required a certain level of status, of course. You had to earn the right to be *that* irresponsible.

Ah, the good old days. Looking back now on my days at the Sydney Futures Exchange, I realize that it was a lot like horse racing. You gambled on what you thought was going to happen next, but in this case it was business organized for generally "responsible" adults who hid behind charts and complicated financial analyses. I found that it was mostly about gut instinct, though, and I had plenty of that. There I was, a teenager, making upwards of seventy thousand dollars a year; it was pretty outrageous. I was hanging out with some very successful financial players who were big personalities and well connected. Being accepted into this club gave me confidence, especially after being knocked around so much in school. Not surprisingly, I dedicated many nights to celebrating my newfound status, investing most of my money in having a great time and making sure everyone around me joined in. This cash-rich adventure quite naturally involved a lot of women, and it certainly helped me cultivate a substantial contingent of potential interested parties, as I could always be relied on to pick up the tab. My apprenticeship as a budding playboy also meant that a lot of my mornings involved facing down massive hangovers. My favorite morning-after cure was a bacon and egg sandwich chased down with a double chocolate milkshake. By the time I hit my twenties things went pretty ballistic.

In my early twenties I was earning hundreds of thousands of dollars a year and living a boom-or-bust life, making tons of money one minute, then losing as much as $80,000 in a day at the horse races. My behavior was equally erratic, and my lifestyle habits were starting to weigh on me, so to speak. By the time I hit twenty-four I was more or less forced to dry out at a fancy healthy spa after humiliating myself and my girlfriend at the time by showing up falling-down-drunk at her lavish, twenty-first birthday party. Ultimately, I did fall over—blacking out is more like it—but not before making a scene involving me bear-hugging her teetotaler father and putting him in a headlock (I was big on headlocks on those days). Apparently, I also rather forcibly challenged him to pound some shots with me. My sister, who was a good friend of my girlfriend's, witnessed the whole episode and informed me the next day that she would disown me if I kept up that kind of misbehavior. That morning, I took a hard look at myself in a full-length mirror and I wasn't proud of what I saw. As I bowed my (pounding) head over the kitchen table in shame, my eyes lit on a gift certificate for a week-long stay at Camp Eden, Australia's premiere health resort at the time,

Camp Eden Health Resort, from their promotional literature: "A place of inspiration created to restore your natural energy, rediscover balance and harmony, enhance your inner beauty, and achieve a real sense of well-being." Believe me, I needed that!

which I'd bought at a charity auction. I decided that instead of giving it away to someone as I had intended, I would use it myself. I made a promise to my sister right then and there that I would clean up my act.

A week later, I arrived at Camp Eden. I was the youngest person there by a couple of decades, at least. Ninety percent of the clientele were women. Normally I would have loved those odds, but most of them were old enough to be my mother and their main interest in me had to do with the possibility of fixing me up with their daughters. It was clearly not my scene! As for the few fellow male inmates, the three I shared a bunk room with were all in their late thirties and early forties, each equipped with classic beer bellies. They looked as if they were about to give birth! Little did I know that twenty years later, I would end up looking just like them!

My next challenge at the fat farm for the wealthy, as I'd begun to think of it, was getting used to micronutrient-rich, vegan food, which tasted like rabbit food to me. Luckily, I'd devoured a couple of meat pies and a large Coke at the airport, so I wasn't immediately starving. The staff were all healthy looking and thin, but initially I somehow judged them creepy, like leaders of a secret cult. Meantime, the stockbroker in me did the numbers on the joint and calculated that shrinking fat people was a lucrative business. That reverie, though, was rudely interrupted by being forced to participate in Tai Chi, which I quickly came to hate. All of this was transpiring as I was coming off my fifteen-Coke-a-day habit and my love affair with *le Big Mac.*

Mother Nature, however, is remarkably consistent and efficient. After three days, I lost all my cravings for junk food. There was no guru who made this happen: there was no cult after all. As it turned out, the staff was not secretly evil. Actually, they were simply healthy, pleasant, and eager to help us get healthy. I even started to enjoy vegan food. True to my boom-or-bust nature, I extended my stay for an extra week. When I left, I felt fantastic.

That new leaf lasted for a full eighteen months, during which time I didn't touch a drop of alcohol and adhered to a strict vegetarian diet. Around that time, things also really started to take off for me professionally. I was making big money via a company I'd started with money I'd earned on the trading floor, as well as a couple of million dollars I'd raised from friends and business contacts. I named the company United Capital Securities. However, in the midst of all this success, I somehow or another lost my health compass once again, reverting quickly to my old habits. My body shape echoed that boom-or-bust nature of mine. When I started the business, I weighed about two hundred pounds. When I sold it thirteen years later I was millions of dollars richer, but I also weighed well over three hundred pounds.

That pretty much sums up my life up until I embarked on the Reboot. I was absolutely obsessed with work, and everything that was done (or not done) was in the service of creating personal wealth. This meant that for the most part, exercise was restricted to some serious elbow work lifting drinks; I ate whatever was convenient, however much I wanted, at the many restaurants around the world I frequented. Periodically, I'd do something drastic to detox and give my system a healthy kick. When I was thirty-four, for example, I read a book by a Qantas Airlines pilot about the health benefits of a "fruitarian" diet, which the author had embarked on after an illness that wasn't being cured by conventional medicine. For one month afterwards I ate only fruits and vegetables. That month cleared out my head and my system and left me feeling great. But following that, I immediately reverted to my usual routine and the yo-yo effect continued until I was forced to really get serious about my health.

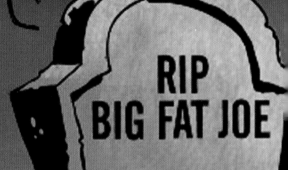

CHAPTER TWO

# GUESS WHO'S COMING TO DINNER? THE GRIM REAPER

PUTTING TOGETHER A DEAL LIKE THIS IS A JUGGLING ACT. ALL THE PIECES HAVE TO LAND IN THE RIGHT PLACE AT THE RIGHT TIME IF IT'S GOING TO WORK.

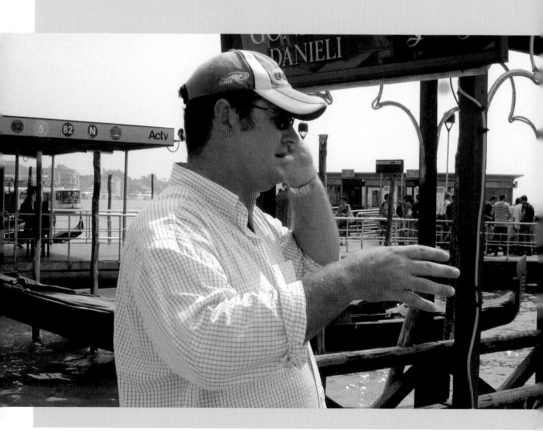

It was the late 1990's, and the Internet bubble was not yet in danger of bursting. I was in my early thirties, and being an entrepreneur, I had at least four or five start-ups on the go. It was an exciting time, to say the least. Vast fortunes were being made overnight, and it seemed as simple to accumulate one as coining a clever word and throwing a "dot com" after it. My expertise was in financial markets, not technology, but I was on fire. I was on the verge of closing out the largest value transaction in my life to date. The deal was worth more than $200 million and it involved a global insurance company, two billionaires, and a hundred employees all being recruited for a new investment bank. The deal had taken me well over twelve months to pull together and had required constant travel to Asia, Europe, the United States, and then back to Australia.

Putting together a deal like this is a juggling act. All the pieces have to land in the right place at the right time if it's going to work out. It was my job to be the juggler, and while I had played that role many times before on other deals, those deals were small potatoes in comparison. I stood to earn quite a bit of money if the venture was successful. In July of 1999, the juggling was over, the deal consummated. I was in Los Angeles at the time, and it was time to celebrate. I treated myself to an expensive set of golf clubs, rented a convertible Mustang, and headed down the 405 with the top down to a Four Seasons resort near San Diego. Life was good.

That's me wheeling and dealing even on holiday in Venice, Italy.

I'd arranged some time with a golf pro on my first day there, and after finishing eighteen holes, I ordered a simple and delicious meal consisting mainly of vegetables to make up for my over-indulgence in the food and drink category over the last few weeks. I went to bed feeling more relaxed than I had in a very long time. However, several hours after falling asleep, I woke up with a strange, tingling sensation all over my body. I switched on the light and saw that my chest and legs were speckled with red, angry-looking welts. I thought perhaps I had poison ivy or some other rash that would soon go away, so I did my best to ignore the whole thing and go back to sleep. By the next morning, the redness had subsided and I went out for another round of golf. That evening, though, the welts returned with more ferocity than before. This time my entire body was covered, including my scalp. My hands and feet became blistery and swollen, getting more and more bloated by the minute. When I looked at myself in the mirror, I remember thinking, "I look like the Elephant Man!" Whatever was going on, I knew it wasn't good. I decided to cut my celebrations short and immediately checked out of the hotel, driving straight to LAX Airport to get the first flight I could back home to Sydney. By this time the welts were so painful that I couldn't even manage to lift my bag into the overhead compartment on the plane. It was the longest, most uncomfortable flight of my life.

I landed in Sydney, and went right to St. Vincent's Hospital and checked in. The medical staff was just as clueless as I was about what was causing my symptoms, but they gave me 60 mg of the steroid Prednisone and the outbreak subsided. Within two or three hours the rash almost completely disappeared. Moreover, the Prednisone gave me a bit of a buzz, as if I had consumed two or three energy drinks in a row. Eight hours later, though, the symptoms returned, so I stayed in the hospital, where I remained under observation for the next two weeks. The doctors continued experimenting with my Prednisone dosage, finding that as soon as they reduced it even slightly, the welts and swelling came back. I underwent a battery of tests over the next fourteen days, during which I nearly went stark raving mad out of restlessness and boredom. But even after all that time and attention, no one could tell me anything other than that I had hives that could only be controlled with Prednisone. They told me the condition was "idiopathic:" in other words, they had no idea what was causing it. I left the hospital with my prescription bottles in hand and very little understanding of how much the drug and the disease itself would impact me over the long term, though I was apprised of the side effects. Prednisone works by essentially knocking out pretty much everything in its path, including my urticaria, but not without causing a lot of collateral damage along the way. It's like the napalm of steroids and used to treat many different problems, such as asthma, various skin diseases, and numerous autoimmune-related problems. As I left the hospital that day in 1999, though, all I cared about was getting back to work and moving on with my life. If I needed Prednisone to make that happen, so be it.

# WHY DID I WANT TO GET OFF PREDNISONE SO BADLY?

Prednisone is a corticosteroid. Corticosteroids mimic the effects of the hormones our bodies produce naturally, and in my case, they worked to reduce the symptoms of my urticaria. How? By suppressing my immune system to help control the way the urticaria was causing my immune system to mistakenly attack itself. So what are the possible down sides to short and long-term Prednisone use? That's where things get sticky:

So you can see why I wanted to get myself off Prednisone!

→ Fluid retention, including swelling in legs and feet

→ Weight gain, with possible buildup of fat deposits

→ Elevated blood pressure

→ Mood swings and depression

→ Insomnia

→ Increased risk of infection

→ Elevated blood sugar, possibly leading to diabetes

→ Loss of calcium, which can lead to osteoporosis and fractures

→ Serious eye problems

→ Cushing's syndrome (or moon face)

I tried, in the ensuing weeks, to tell myself that the urticaria was actually a short-term anomaly and not a chronic condition, but after a few months of symptoms, I resigned myself to the fact that it was the new reality. I was depressed about it, but also determined not to let it really get me down.

What was my new normal? First of all, it was always being on enough Prednisone to be able to live a "normal" life. I found out that outbreaks could be triggered by even the slightest human contact, such as a handshake or a hug. Just the pressure of gripping a golf club could bring on an attack, as could wearing a backpack, walking on a sandy beach without shoes, or, for that matter, wearing shoes. I couldn't use an exercise bike at the gym because of the pressure from the seat. Sitting for hours on an airplane was now always excruciating, since the weight of my body on the seat put pressure on my skin, which in turn triggered an outbreak. Attacks could be set off by a lack of sleep, or by sunlight. The physical act of sex became more of a negotiation than a pleasure because the pressure involved could produce a painful outbreak. Girlfriends had to embrace my "low impact" playbook. I remember being glad that my business didn't involve any heavy lifting or manual labor, as that would have completely ruined me.

One particularly frightening outbreak occurred when I was still very much in denial about the seriousness of my condition.

Before I got sick I used to love getting massages—I still do. After I got sick and massages became more problematic because of the pressure involved, I would always warn the masseuse not to do deep tissue work on me, but every now and then I would still push it and tempt fate because the deep tissue massages felt so good. On one particular occasion, I was having a massage and the masseuse was doing some work on my abdomen, which was particularly tense. At the time, it felt great, and I left the table feeling very relaxed. From there, I rushed off to a tennis match with a girl I was dating at the time, who was named Jemma.

By the way, talking about my condition was not something I often did at that time, particularly when it came to conversations with girls on dates. But on this occasion, I was sitting at the Sydney Olympic Tennis Stadium next to Jemma and was starting to feel some worrisome after-effects from the deep tissue massage. I could detect histamines being released into my stomach, and my body starting to go into shock. Looking back on this now, I realize that for the eight years during which my urticaria was in full bloom, the outbreak that day at the tennis stadium was the worst by far. I was experiencing excruciating stomach cramps, to the point where I wasn't sure I could stand the pain. I told Jemma what was going on and naturally, she wanted to call an ambulance, but I asked her if she could just get me home to my precious Prednisone. I was worried about the seriousness of the attack and whether I could make it all the way home, but at the same time, I knew the drill: an ambulance would show up, the EMS workers would administer a shot of cortisone which was standard operating procedure in such cases, and I would still be in horrific pain. Going to a nearby drugstore for some Prednisone wasn't an option, either. You can't just ask a pharmacist to hand over a dosage of Prednisone; it's too powerful a drug. I had to get home to my stash. We got to the car and Jemma drove. I was starting to feel like I was drifting in and out of consciousness, but we finally got to my apartment just in the nick of time. I took a dosage of Prednisone, and then passed out for the next twelve hours. Jemma sat next to my bed and watched me, fearing that I would deteriorate further. By the next morning, I was feeling better, but it wasn't exactly my idea of a perfect date.

I don't know if words alone can sufficiently explain how completely debilitating this disease has been for me. Its physical and mental toll has been so complex and wide-ranging that most of the time it was easier to suffer through it in silence than to admit how truly sick I was. I was a professional and financial success, but I was also tipping the scales at 300-plus pounds and taking an increasing number of prescription drugs, led by the Prednisone. My mind and soul were as much of a mess as my body, and I was more and more cognizant of the fact that there was no balance in my life. This is what the whole "hitting bottom" thing is about. My extreme nature had finally caught up with me. I had achieved financial success. I had pulled off big deals in the boardroom. I'd started companies from scratch and yet in health terms, I felt as powerless and defenseless as a boy in a bubble. When I looked in the mirror, I didn't even recognize who was staring back at me anymore. I looked fifteen years older than I was. I had the kind of gut I'd seen on my roommates at Camp Eden, and boy, wasn't I sick of people looking down at my stomach, winking, and asking me when the twins were due.

As many times as my extreme personality has gotten me into trouble, I have to admit that it is also a saving grace. It's what enables me to become very single-minded, particularly when it comes to my own survival. I just refused to stop believing that there was an answer out there somewhere, even if no one had yet found it. I had one clue that I hung on to, one observation that offered a possible insight into the puzzle that was my condition. After nights of over-indulging in food and alcohol, it was clear that my outbreaks became worse. The two things had to be related. I began to suspect that what I put into my body had caused the disease and the solution might be equally straightforward. "You are what you eat," right? Well, if that were true, I'd better commit to healing my body in the best way I *knew*—logically, and in my gut (as huge as it was)—I could.

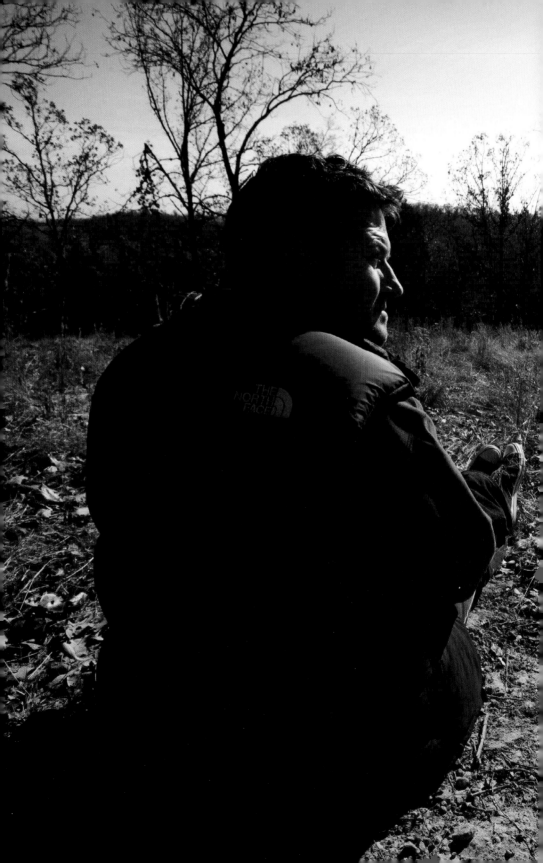

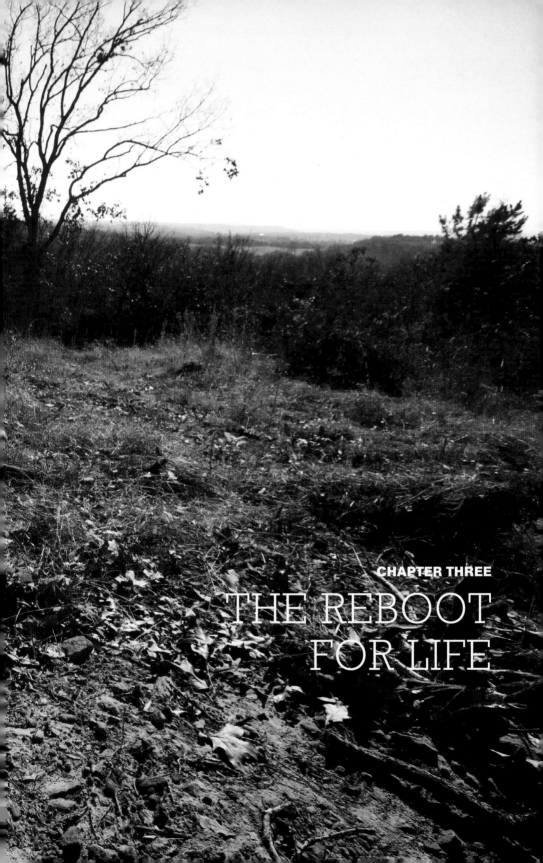

CHAPTER THREE

# THE REBOOT
# FOR LIFE

# IF YOU GO ON A JUICE REBOOT AND HAVE THE GUTS TO TURN UP AT A DINNER PARTY WITH A FLASK OF GREEN JUICE IN HAND, GET READY TO DEFEND YOURSELF...

### LEADING CAUSES OF DEATH IN THE U.S.

| | | | |
|---|---|---|---|
| 1. | Heart Disease | 631,636 | 26% |
| 2. | Cancer | 559,888 | 23% |
| 3. | Stroke | 137,119 | 6% |
| 4. | Chronic Respiratory | 124,583 | 5% |
| 5. | Accidents | 121,599 | 5% |
| 6. | Alzheimer's | 72,449 | 3% |
| 7. | Diabetes | 72,432 | 3% |
| 8. | Influenza / Pneumonia | 56,326 | 2% |
| 9. | Nephritis | 45,344 | 2% |
| 10. | Septicemia | 34,234 | 1% |

### COST OF ILLNESS IN THE U.S. ($B)

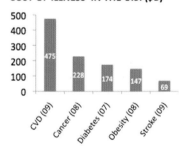

### % OF OBESE IN THE U.S.

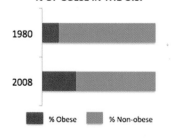

### % OF OVERWEIGHT AND OBESE IN THE U.S.

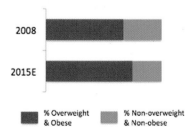

There is no way around it: deciding to go on an all-juice Reboot is a radical thing to do. It's like a mini-protest, as if you are saying: "I am going to take a five, ten, thirty (or sixty!)-day hiatus from regular society." It means when you sit down to a business lunch, you are restricting your intake to a glass of fresh juice instead of whatever meal your colleagues are partaking of. It means sidelining your usual routines and rituals, such as your morning coffee and bagel, or the glass of wine that marks the end of your working day. Taken separately, these seem like easy things to give up, but when you scratch them all off your list at the same time, you've done something pretty extreme. Truthfully, it's one of the reasons I love doing it so much. As the CEO of my investment firm and a board member of several other companies, it's one of the few truly subversive things I get to do these days.

It is in this spirit of rebellion that I warn you: if you go on a juice Reboot and have the guts to turn up at a dinner party with a flask of green juice in hand, get ready to defend yourself, because you will be judged. And also prepare for most of the conversation throughout the night to center on what people do and don't eat, and what's good for you and what's not. Everybody's an expert. Everybody has an opinion. Most of the time you just get people saying (or looking at you as if to say): "Joe! That can't be good for you. Are you crazy?!"

Why now? It's simple: The facts on obesity and illness are grim

source: The Centers for Disease Control and Prevention (CDC)

To them, my answer is, "maybe." But perhaps not as crazy as you might think, thank you very much. What the naysayers don't realize is that I'm not talking about some fad diet you'd read about in a magazine. What I'm doing is applying the principles of an ancient tradition—one that straddles millennia and diverse cultures—to my own life, right here in the 21st century.

The principles behind the Reboot are rooted firmly in the practice of fasting, which has a long and venerable role in the history of humankind. Fasting, whether via juicing or in a more extreme form, goes about as far back as you can imagine. For example, in North America, many Native Americans thought of fasting as a sacred custom. As a coming-of-age rite, young boys got sent off into the wilderness on "vision quests" in which they would fast in order to gain spiritual wisdom.

There are countless references to fasting in the Bible, where it was usually conducted as a means of repenting, lamenting, or seeking wisdom or clarity. Jesus fasted for forty days and forty nights. Moses and David also fasted. An early Christian belief held that Satan gained entrance to a person's soul through the ingesting of food, so fasting was a way of purifying the body, gaining humility, and getting closer to God. Later, fasting continued to be used as an expression of sacrifice and devotion during periods such as Lent, or other holy days.

On one of the holiest days in Judaism, Yom Kippur, or the Day of Atonement, observers abstain from eating and drinking as they ask for forgiveness for promises they've broken. During the Islamic holy month of Ramadan, believers fast during the day and then eat only one small meal in the evening. Hindus and Buddhists fast as a means of purification.

Plato, Socrates, Pythagoras—even Hippocrates, the father of Western medicine—these wisest of men are known to have regularly fasted for improved mental and physical efficiency. Pythagoras routinely fasted for up to forty days at a time. Hippocrates not only fasted himself, but often prescribed fasting to his patients, as did the great physician Paracelsus.

Perhaps the most renowned modern practitioner of the fast was Mahatma Gandhi, the pioneer of India's independence born in 1869. Gandhi didn't fast merely to benefit his own health, or for spiritual gain. He used fasting as a nonviolent method of affecting change via "passive resistance." Ghandi conducted at least fourteen fasts of varying lengths in his lifetime that were also political acts. When not fasting, he maintained a vegetarian diet, later becoming more of a self-described fruitarian. He, too, liked the increased clarity and energy he felt from eating what I call "first-tier" foods, by which I mean foods grown in the earth and nourished by the sun.

Fasting can be defined as intentionally abstaining from food or from eating certain foods for a purpose that is productive. For some, this might mean drinking only water for a finite period. For my purposes, fasting meant ingesting only fruit and vegetable juices, as well as water, for a pre-determined amount of time. What did this mean for my body? It

# BENEFITS OF FASTING*

INCREASED ENERGY AND VITALITY

IMPROVED IMMUNE FUNCTION

IMPROVED HAIR, SKIN, NAILS

INCREASED CLARITY, MEMORY, FOCUS

INCREASED JOINT FLEXIBILITY

FEWER MOOD SWINGS/ DEPRESSION LIFTS

FEELING CALMER

IMPROVED VISION AND HEARING

INCREASED REGULARITY

INCREASED STAMINA

CHRONIC DISEASE SYMPTOMS REDUCED OR ERADICATED

AN INCREASED SENSE OF OPTIMISM

WOW!

*These were Joe's experiences, yours may be different.

meant that during that time it wasn't required to use so much energy breaking down difficult-to-digest foods, i.e., meat, dairy products, refined sugars, caffeine, white flour (by the way, technically, white flour by itself is easy to digest, but junk foods made with it are not), and the like, so it could use that extra energy for the purpose of self-healing. Fasting offers a physiological break to the digestive tract and central nervous system. Normally, the body is continually working to digest food, to eliminate waste, to battle disease and resist sickness, to replenish cells and enrich and nourish the blood. But if there is less to digest, and we are eating easier-to-digest, "first-tier" foods such as fruits and vegetables, the body only requires a minimum amount of energy to support its other functions.

Ironically, I'd first heard about the benefits of fasting when I was a trader on the futures exchange in Sydney. Those guys weren't looking for a spiritual transformation or anything like that. Their motivation was purely monetary, to gain an edge on the trading floor by having their minds crystal clear. The idea sort of appealed to me, and I had to admit that my lunchtime Chinese meal chased down by beer did make me feel drowsy, but I always countered the feeling by drinking five or six cans of Coke. In any case, I loved food too much to give it up for clarity or any other reason.

It wasn't until many years later, after traversing the peaks and valleys of my weight gains and losses—and the onset of my urticaria and subsequent prescription drug reliance—that I really started doing my homework on the subject. That is when I learned about the biological science behind fasting and why it enables a person's entire being to be re-energized. How did it also work to lessen the effects of my urticaria? Fasting greatly reduces the immune system's workload by sparing our digestive tracts some work, particularly from dealing with the inflammation that is often caused by allergic reactions to processed foods, sugars, grains, and proteins. It's clear to me that inflammation is at the root of so many chronic diseases. Inflammation is not natural. Some inflammation is necessary and natural—like when we get a cut—because our bodies need this process to live. Excessive inflammation from too much junk food and other environmental factors is not "natural" or healthy. The word "inflammation" itself suggests that something is wrong, that something from outside the body is invading and provoking a reaction. If it is true that the trigger for inflammation is due to an outside source, it's likely that the cause is something we are ingesting via food or drink.

The fluids in our bodies have what's called a pH level. In chemistry, pH is a measure of how acidic or how alkaline a solution or substance is. Pure water, for example, is said to be neutral, with a pH value of around seven. Solutions with a pH of less than seven are considered acidic, while those of more than seven are considered alkaline. The food we eat and the liquid we drink have an effect on our systems that is either alkaline or acidic. If we eat food that reduces our pH levels and tends to be more acidic, it means that our systems are breeding grounds for inflammation. The more alkaline our diets, the opposite is true. No prizes for guessing in which category fruits and vegetables belong. (The concept of being able to alter our blood pH via diet is hotly contested and not yet scientifically proven—there are still varying opinions on the issue. But it makes sense to me!)

On a deeper level, fasting is thought to promote cell rejuvenation first by reducing serum fats in our blood, which thins the blood and allows more oxygen to reach the tissues; then, by mobilizing and releasing toxins stored in our fat, the process in turn promotes healthy cell generation. After a period of time on a juice Reboot, your body goes into a state known as ketosis, triggering the body to turn stored fat into energy.

The body contains about two hundred different cell types. As our 100 trillion or so cells routinely die off or become damaged, new ones form. For most of us, only about half our cells are working in peak condition at any given time. Many people believe that diseases occur within us because our cells are saturated by toxins, and thus can't effectively resist disease the way the immune system could if all our cells were healthy and functioning properly. It is our poor diets and our sedentary lifestyles that slow down our metabolisms, render our digestive processes less efficient, and deprive our cells of key nutrients, thereby exacerbating the process of cellular degeneration and decay. Simply

# SPECIAL REPORT FROM THE FRONT LINES OF CANCER RESEARCH

In 2007, the World Cancer Research Fund with the American Institute for Cancer Research completed a five-year study for which leading scientists from around the world worked together to come up with recommendations for how people could reduce their risk of cancer via food, nutrition, and physical activity.

In a nutshell, here is what they came up with:

**1** Be as lean as possible within your normal range of body weight, aiming for a BMI (body mass index) of 18.5-25

**2** Get between thirty and sixty minutes of physical activity a day

**3** Limit your consumption of "energy-dense," processed foods and avoid sugary drinks—drink lots of water!

**4** Eat a diet made up mainly of plant food—at least five servings a day of fruits and vegetables

**5** Limit your intake of red meat and avoid processed meats

**6** Limit your alcohol consumption

**7** Limit your salt intake

**8** Don't count on dietary supplements for "nutritional adequacy"

put, fasting or "rebooting" the system helps to eliminate dead and dying cells while encouraging the generation of new ones.

It takes just a day on a Reboot for this process to kick in, since it is within the first twenty-four hours that certain digestive enzymes stop entering the stomach. Instead, other enzymes are released into the intestines and the bloodstream, where they circulate to digest waste and destroy dead, diseased, and damaged cells without harming the healthy ones.

I'd learned a lot about myself during my previous Rebooting attempts and discovered firsthand some fundamental truths about the power of the human body, as well as the power I had over it. Know thyself—good idea. Know thy cells—even better! So…what happened to all that self-empowerment?

Honestly, in my previous efforts I'd never been willing to fully commit to a junk-food-and-booze-free lifestyle. My food addictions kept getting in the way of Mother Nature's natural healing process. Truth be told, I was sleeping with the enemy, albeit mostly only on weekends. I tried to limit my temptations by hiring Millie Katter, one of Sydney's best nutritional chefs. She came to my office every weekday and cooked beautiful, healthy lunches. Putting Millie in charge of my kitchen was a brilliant idea, until I started cheating on her. I would quite often have a hangover in the mornings, so I'd pick up an egg and bacon roll and a can of Coke to steady the ship before she arrived. I would eat my lovingly prepared lunch and then splurge on a decadent dinner, or spend the night in front of the television with a couple of bars of chocolate and some ice cream. I was always careful to hide the packaging, limiting the evidence of my nutritional crimes.

Additionally, going to spas, eating vegetarian, and giving up alcohol for months at a time were part of my quick-fix strategy, they weren't about long-term solutions. The reward for being on such a restricted diet was always a meal of all my favorite things at the end. There was always a cheeseburger waiting for me, a case of Cokes in the refrigerator, and ice cream in the freezer. Crazy as it may sound, it was the reward of junk food that kept me off the junk food: the paradox of a boom-or-bust life.

I tell you all this because it will help you understand why I finally undertook this massive jump. There was a kind of rhythm to my eating patterns. I ate and drank whatever I wanted most of the time, then put myself on a fruit-and-vegetable-only diet for a month or so, after which I could go right back to how I ate before. At that point, my number one priority remained work, and not what was good long-term for Joe Cross; I clearly wasn't ready to make the commitment that that kind of change would entail. As a result, my weight fluctuated wildly and I realized that I was like a car with only two speeds: flat-out indulgence, eating and drinking everything in sight with a lot of cigarettes along the way; or doing a cleanse to detox, then going right back to the starting line. There was no middle road.

I had not yet resolved within myself that in order for me to conquer my disease permanently, I would have to adhere to a total nutritional overhaul and sever my relationship with my favorite foods. I needed to put an end, once and for all, to my literally suicidal behavior with food. I could not afford any more slip-ups, birthday treats, or late night pizza calls when drunk. In fact, being drunk had to go as well. Though all of my vices could leave knowing they were once very dear to me, our time together was officially over. Having the best of both worlds just wasn't working for me, so I made the decision to choose life over death, or more specifically, greens over grease!

Why would this time be different? Because I had made the commitment to do whatever it would take to cure my disease and be drug-free, starting with a sixty-day, all-juice Reboot. I knew it would be a radical undertaking, but the situation with my disease had reached a tipping point. Something inside me said: "Joe: it's now or never." I didn't have all the answers before setting off on the Reboot, but I believed that the process would guide me to a place where the truth would be revealed, and that truth would set me free. In this regard, the entire endeavor required a leap of faith. So, I took a large one.

On top of that, I was going public with the whole experience by choosing to make a film about it. There would be no hiding out after this. Rise or fall, I would be in the spotlight and it would be recorded for all to see. There was no doubt that two months of juicing would be tough, but for my body to heal itself, I felt that it would require me to go deep into the process.

Before I left Australia for New York, where I intended to begin my journey, I had some photographs taken of me with my shirt off. What I saw was a huge, round belly that made it tough for me to get around without an expenditure of effort nearly as great as the mound of flesh itself. When I first set eyes on those pictures they were shocking. I guess I hadn't fully realized what 300 or so pounds looked like on me, and it wasn't pretty. I looked like I'd swallowed a sheep. I stored those photos away on my iPhone to remind me where I'd been, and where I wanted to go.

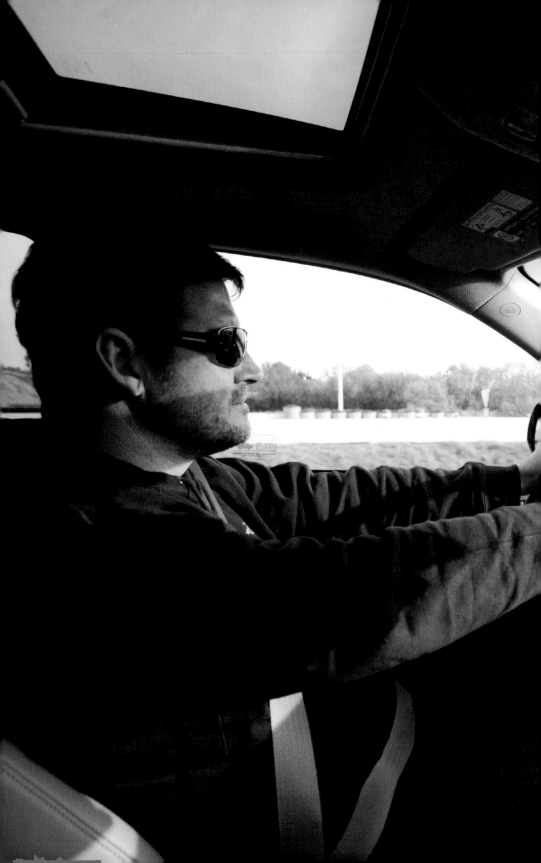

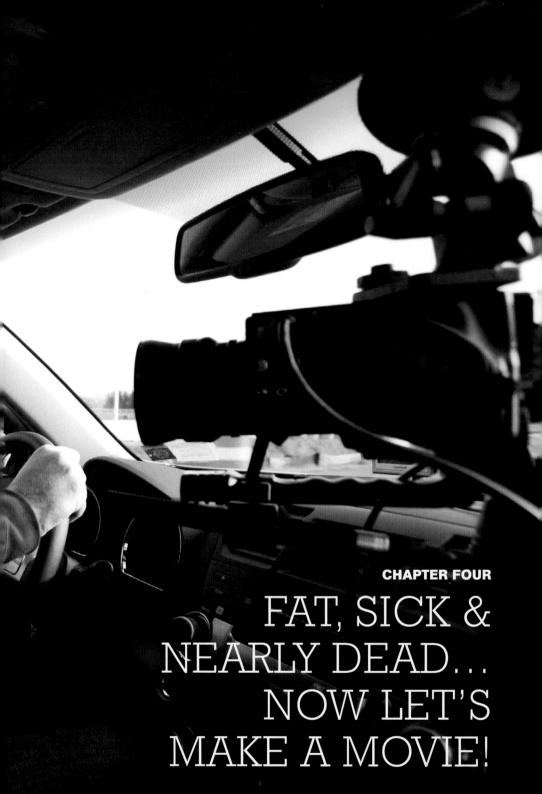

# CHAPTER FOUR

# FAT, SICK & NEARLY DEAD... NOW LET'S MAKE A MOVIE!

I VIEWED THE WHOLE PROJECT AS A POTENTIALLY LIFE-SAVING SCIENCE EXPERIMENT IN WHICH I WAS LEAD SPECIMEN AND SOLE PATRON.

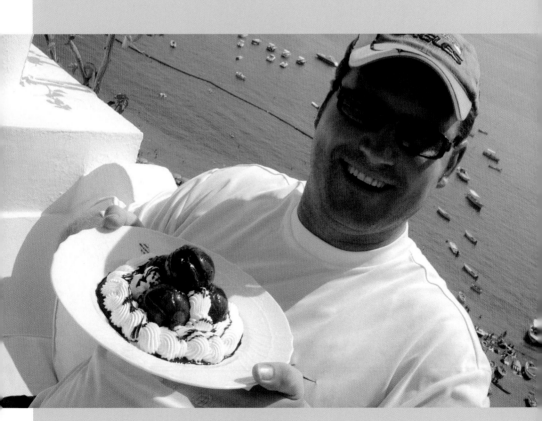

As committed as I now was to the Reboot and to making the film, the weeks before I left Sydney that led up to it were not my finest. Instead of properly preparing for a full two months of consuming only juice by gradually moderating my diet, which all experts recommend, I had been binging like there was no tomorrow. I don't know whether this was me wanting to cling to old habits, having a last hurrah with all my old vices, or just me doing things the way I'd always done them—to the extreme. In any case, I managed to gain a few extra pounds and my urticaria was at its most severe. From experience, I knew this would make getting things back under control even more difficult.

I landed in New York and checked into my hotel in Manhattan's meatpacking district. As I sat in my room that night with just a few hours to go before the film crew arrived to pick me up in the wee hours of the morning, I couldn't help wondering what I was getting myself into. For a start, I'd never been in front of a camera before and had no idea whether or not I'd be any good at it. I knew I could be counted on to tell a good story at a dinner party, but even that was usually with a few glasses of wine under my belt.

I'd have to hope that my storytelling skills would stay with me in front of the camera *sans* wine and absent the dinner companions, and that the innate drama of my story would be powerful enough to satisfy an audience, or at least to make my mother proud. The "dramatic" premise was: *for sixty days, a fat, rich guy confesses his lifelong weaknesses— among them the junk food addictions that are literally killing him—to anyone who will listen, while at the same time carting around a mysterious, dark green juice that is so powerful it leaves a permanent moustache stain around his mouth.*

Hmmm. I was beginning to sense that the inherent drama of the story might not do the trick either...Maybe I should just focus on looking really good in front of the camera. Okay, here we go, take two: *A rich, fat guy who looks really good in front of the camera but lives for two months on green, swampy juice while journeying across America in a blue Toyota, fueled by his hunger for the truth about fruits and vegetables (and also by his hunger)...*

On paper, this would be a very tough film "treatment" to sell to Hollywood. As someone who has made a living putting together deals for investors, my instincts told me this one would not be an easy sell, which is why I was making it with my own money, as well as with financial contributions from a few mates who wanted to lend support.

Why was I taking this personal and financial risk? I viewed the whole project as a potentially life-saving science experiment in which I was lead specimen and sole patron. At the center of the venture was a sincere desire to free myself from my illness and prescription drug reliance, and to prove something I already believed in: that the human body can cure itself of most things if it is nourished in the right way. So instead of giving a chunk of money to a scientific foundation that would employ a team of white coats to poke and prod this idea under a microscope and reward my patronage with an invite to their annual cocktail party, I'd decided to go it alone and perform the experiment myself, on myself. In this respect the film crew would be my peer review, the camera the microscope. And perhaps, in the process, we might also come up with a good movie.

What was the worst-case scenario? I would get to see a bit of the United States, I would form some healthier eating habits and other routines, and only my Mom would like the film. But even *she* would insist on one thing: I should stick with the plan until I was cured!

That night in my room I couldn't stop looking at the clock. I was already hungry and it was only 10:00 pm—still two hours until the Reboot officially began. I tried to distract myself by reflecting on how I'd gotten myself involved in this thing.

I'd first met Robert Mac, a documentary filmmaker and writer from Sydney, while he was looking for investors for a new project of his own. Turning the tables on him, I announced that I had an idea for a movie. I told him I wanted to make a film about fasting. Robert was intrigued. I don't think he'd pegged me for the sort of bloke who knew anything about a topic like fasting, since the idea didn't exactly seem like the kind of thought that would spring from the mind of a tall, heavy, extroverted guy who was at the time the President of the Manly Rugby League Football

Club, a celebrated institution dedicated to brawn, biffo, and playing the toughest contact sport on the planet. But as counterintuitive as it may have initially seemed to Robert, I had in fact become a bit of an expert in this area through my own research and experimentation, and via chats I'd had with medical types, including my father and brother.

Once I'd explained all about my illness to Robert, he was hooked. It didn't take much convincing, in truth, as Robert had done fasts himself and understood the biological science behind it. Also, fasting complemented Robert's life as a yogi, a world in which fasting is thought of as a spiritual ritual to rest the body and restore vitality. He believed, as I did, that I probably could cure myself if I fasted for long enough. He urged me, "Tell the truth about this, Joe, and the world will listen. They wouldn't believe it coming from someone like me because I look like a hippie."

Robert followed up our initial meeting with a proposal for us to work together on this shared passion, and from there the project began to take shape. I put Robert on the payroll and he became my co-creator and executive producer. For about a year leading up to the shoot we prepared a schedule, and while we didn't always see eye-to-eye on how best to tell the story, our healthy debate continued for several years until the project was complete. There would be many twists and turns along the way, including a chance meeting in Winslow, Arizona that would completely change the direction of the film.

The clock was still ticking away slowly in my hotel room. There was still an hour to go until midnight. I was both excited and nervous, but I trusted the one part of myself I knew I could always count on: my gut. I mean that in a strictly metaphorical sense. But speaking of guts, I decided to give in to my last-minute urge for some comfort food. I went out and ordered a cheeseburger and a chocolate milkshake from an all-night, good old-fashioned American diner. I felt a little guilty about it, but it was delicious. I hoped, though, that it would be my last slip-up for a long time. I went back to the hotel and drifted off to sleep.

At 6 a.m. sharp I received a wake-up call. I got right out of bed, showered, and hurried downstairs to meet the film crew, who were waiting for me outside in the van. We would have to hurry if we were going to make it out to our first stop to see Dr. Joel Fuhrman, whose offices were in Flemington, New Jersey.

Dr. Fuhrman, who had agreed to monitor me on the Reboot, is among the U.S.'s leading medical experts in the field of nutritional health. Flemington is about an hour outside New York City, so we headed through the Holland Tunnel and west on Route 78. All around me in the van were people eating bagels and drinking coffee, and as I got settled I realized we'd forgotten something very important: my juice! We were not off to a good start.

Dr. Fuhrman has treated more than ten thousand patients over the course of his career, most of whom have landed in his office after years of being overweight, chronically ill, and unhappy as a result. Some of them are extremely sick and desperate by the time they land on his doorstep. More often than not, those patients, like me, have tried countless diets and other methods to lose weight and get healthy, but to no avail; they have lost and regained weight many times and no diet has stuck. They are at the end of their ropes. They are diabetic and tired of being dependent on insulin or dialysis. They have been told they need heart bypass surgery, and are desperate to find another way to get healthy that doesn't involve an invasive, life-threatening procedure. For these patients, as for me, the goal is to lose weight. But just as importantly, it's to find some way of not being dependent on prescription medication for the rest of their lives, of helping their bodies to heal through the adoption of healthy nutritional practices.

We've all heard of calories. Calories refer to a measurement of energy. If something has 100 calories, it has twice the amount of energy as something with 50 calories. But energy can come in different forms. Dr. Fuhrman's notion is that you can consume foods that provide energy and contain high nutritional value, or you can consume foods that have energy but little nutritional value. A good example is a fast-food burger whose calorie count is 600 or so, vs. 600 calories worth of broccoli. Both of these foods contain the same amount of energy, or calories, but the broccoli offers about one hundred times more nutritional value than the burger. Another way of looking at it is that you would need to eat one hundred burgers to get as much nutrition as you would from one bowl of

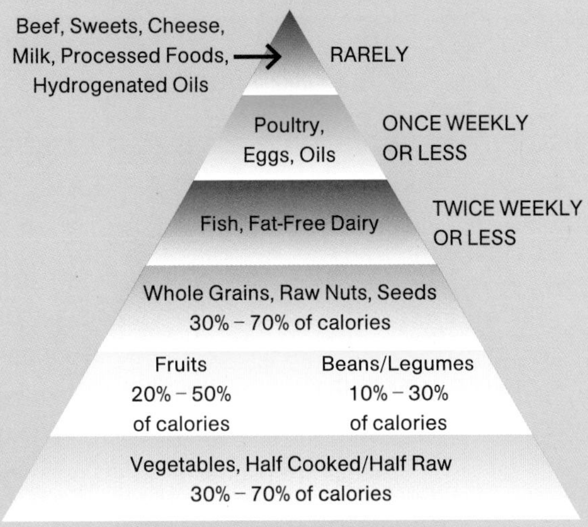

Beef, Sweets, Cheese, Milk, Processed Foods, Hydrogenated Oils
RARELY
Poultry, Eggs, Oils
ONCE WEEKLY OR LESS
Fish, Fat-Free Dairy
TWICE WEEKLY OR LESS
Whole Grains, Raw Nuts, Seeds
30% – 70% of calories
Fruits
20% – 50% of calories
Beans/Legumes
10% – 30% of calories
Vegetables, Half Cooked/Half Raw
30% – 70% of calories


Dr. Fuhrman's Food Pyramid turns the way we usually eat on its head. Here is his recommendation

www.drfuhrman.com



# DR. FUHRMAN'S NUTRIENT DENSITY SCORES

A large assortment of micronutrients are considered in the scoring totals present in an equal caloric portion of each food, with special attention paid to micronutrients with known anti-cancer potential. For more information about calculation methods see DrFuhrman.com

| | | | | | | | |
|---|---|---|---|---|---|---|---|
| Mustard Greens | 100 | Onions | 30 | Cucumber | 11 | Low-Fat Plain | |
| Watercress | 100 | Cherries | 28 | Pomegranate | | Yogurt | 2 |
| Kale | 100 | Grapes | 27 | Juice | 10 | Whole Wheat Bread | 2 |
| Turnip Greens | 100 | Strawberries | 27 | Sweet Potato | 10 | Olive Oil | 2 |
| Collard Greens | 100 | Mushrooms | 27 | Tofu | 10 | Apple Juice | 1 |
| Brussels Sprouts | 90 | Tomato | 25 | Apple | 9 | White Bread | 1 |
| Bok Choy | 85 | Sesame Seeds | 23 | Pistachio Nuts | 9 | Chicken Breast | 1 |
| Spinach | 81 | Blueberries | 19 | Green Peas | 8 | Eggs | 1 |
| Arugula | 76 | Sunflower Seeds | 18 | Avocado | 7 | White Pasta | 1 |
| Cauliflower | 60 | Artichoke | 18 | Cashews | 6 | Shrimp | 1 |
| Cabbage | 55 | Walnuts | 18 | Mango | 6 | Ground Beef, | |
| Romaine | 52 | Orange | 18 | Peanut Butter | 6 | 85% lean | -4 |
| Broccoli | 46 | Cantaloupe | 14 | Corn | 5 | Feta Cheese | -5 |
| Asparagus | 42 | Peaches | 13 | Bananas | 4 | Low-Fat Cheddar | |
| Flax Seeds | 37 | Kidney Beans | 12 | Brown Rice | 4 | Cheese | -6 |
| Carrots | 35 | Lentils | 12 | Oatmeal | 4 | Potato Chips | -9 |
| Green Bell | | Edamame | 11 | White Potato | 3 | French Fries | -9 |
| Pepper | 34 | Iceburg Lettuce | 11 | Salmon | 2 | Vanilla Ice Cream | -9 |
| Almonds | 30 | Pineapple | 11 | Skim Milk | 2 | Cola | -10 |

broccoli. That is why Dr. Fuhrman promotes a "nutrient-dense" diet. He tells his patients that food supplies us with nutrients and calories. The calories come from carbohydrates, fats, and proteins, while nutrients are byproducts of non-caloric food factors such as vitamins, minerals, fiber, and phytochemicals (or phytonutrients), which are essential to our health. To maintain health, including a healthy weight level, we must *eat a preponderance of food with a high proportion of nutrients to calories.*

I have a theory based on gut instinct, not science, that one of the reasons, when you eat processed foods like that burger, that you feel hungry again just an hour or so later is because the burger didn't have much to offer in the first place in terms of nutritive value. Our bodies crave nutrition and force our bodies to keep eating until they get enough of it. So when you eat food that is high in nutritive value, you can actually eat less and be more satisfied than when you eat foods that are high calorie, low nutritional value foods. (And by the way, it turns out that science does prove this to be true.)

Simply put, Dr. Fuhrman is a guy who knows what he's doing and believes passionately that healthy eating can cure us from most diseases. I knew he would help me keep focused during the course of my Reboot. The crew and I got out of the car and carried our equipment up two flights to his office.

He weighed me in at 308 pounds. He took my blood pressure and measured my body/fat ratio, as well as my electrolyte level. The plan was that he would be keeping an eye on my blood test results, including electrolytes and my other vitals, throughout the Reboot process.

While we were there, we also conducted an interview with him for the film. By the time we captured what we needed and completed my evaluations, the day was just about over. I was cranky and exhausted, having gone the entire time without the juices I was supposed to be drinking at regular intervals. I was truly starving and feeling very low on energy. We left New Jersey and headed all the way out to Long Island, to the Hamptons, which is about three or four hours in the other direction. The idea was that for the next week I would stay there in a house borrowed from some friends, where I could take it easy and begin to get my sea legs during the tough first days of the juice Reboot. I knew the detoxifica-

The most precious commodity we
have is time, which greatly increases
in value if we are healthy and happy.

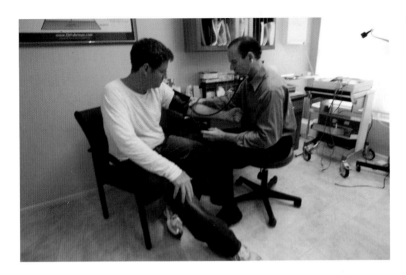

Me, getting
checked out by
Dr. Fuhrman.

tion process would leave me feeling extremely tired, and I planned to just hunker down and let it do its cleansing work.

That evening, I finally got my juice and settled into the house in the Hamptons. It was large, and I was alone in it. I was a very long way from my family and friends in Australia, who were at that very moment enjoying the summer festivities in Sydney, though it was a cold October night in New York. It was the end of Day One and I had a whopping headache, terrible stomach cramps, and overall felt shot to pieces.

I was about as irritable as it gets, and felt so distracted I couldn't sit still. By the way, this isn't at all unusual during the first few days of a Reboot, when the body is working hard to detoxify, deal with not having caffeine (if you typically drink it), beginning to break certain eating habits, and so on. All I wanted to do was mope and feel sorry for myself. On top of this, the film crew was with me, documenting my self-pity party. So I did what any self-respecting man in his forties would do under these circumstances: I called my Mom, who said all the right things. After that I went to bed, pulled the covers over my head, and went to sleep.

When I woke up the next morning (Day Two), I was still feeling very lethargic, anxious, and headache-y. A question posed by my very curious film crew was: "Why Reboot on juice?"

Juice is digested very rapidly and requires a smaller expenditure of energy than solid food, which gives the body additional time and energy to rid itself of toxins and other unwanted materials it has absorbed. The reason juice works so much better for this purpose is that all the essential ingredients locked within the fibers of fruits and vegetables are freed during the juice extraction process, which means those nutrients can be quickly absorbed and used directly. The digestive system then has to expend only a minimal effort to process the food it is taking in, so much more metabolic energy can be used to cleanse mucoid matter from the lymph system and toxins from cellular tissue.

Knowing what is transpiring physically during a juice cleanse, it makes complete sense that when you start you are going to feel the whole thing is very isolating, as well as physically and psychologically challenging.

Think about when you or someone you know first quit smoking, for example. Most people complain they initially notice all sorts of symptoms they didn't even have when they were smoking two packs a day, such as increased coughing, expelling mucous from the lungs, muscle pain, dark circles under the eyes, and insomnia. These symptoms frequently last weeks after the last cigarette. Now, common sense might prompt the question: if cigarettes are bad for me, why is it that I feel worse when I stop smoking? The answer is that since you have given your body the chance, it is attempting to detoxify itself by flushing out those poisons via the blood, the lymph system, excretions, etc., to begin the process of regeneration. That is how the body heals itself.

When you embark on a juice Reboot, you are super-charging this healing process and, initially, this is one of the toughest things about it. One theory is that the body uses the juice as an opportunity to flush out its 100 trillion cells or, in other words, to *detoxify*. Sometimes, this will show up in the form of headaches, cold or flu-like symptoms, coughing, feelings of gassiness or bloating, fatigue or insomnia, skin breakouts, constipation or diarrhea, thirst, bad breath—all of which happened with me. Even my dreams were affected.

This exchange of the old for the new may not be noticeable or dramatic for everyone, and depends in large part on what your diet was like

Would I be able to live a normal life, or would I be sidelined to one where getting out of my car or sitting in an airplane seat would be an ordeal?

before the Reboot, and how many toxins need to escape the system. These symptoms are a body's way of saying goodbye to all that crap. When you burn off metabolic waste in this way it is actually a good thing. If we don't do this periodically, we end up retaining waste in our cells. And that, my friends, is what can lead to disease.

You must realize that I hadn't come to this crossroads because I'd sat around thinking: "Joe, if you keep up your bad habits you are going to die young." I don't even think we humans are coded to think that way about life and death—it's just not something we can process realistically and still go on about our daily business. But we do spend a lot of time thinking about our hopes and dreams for the future, whether these entail meeting a soul mate, having a family, starting a business, or traveling around the world.

Most of our aspirations involve mobility and wellness, so that when we do meet potential soul mates, they see a future with us that is not limited by illness. When we raise a family, we need to be able to toss a ball around, carry kids in our arms. When we start a business, we need to show up at the office looking ready for action, ready to take on the world. For many of us, vacationing in exotic locations like pristine beaches or foreign cities is one of the things we dream we will do when the kids are a little older, when there's a little more cash in the bank.

All of these dreams and more were what particularly scared me when it came to thinking about my weight, the urticaria, and Prednisone. Would I be able to live a normal life, or would I be sidelined to one where getting out of my car or sitting in an airplane seat would be an ordeal? I couldn't live with the idea that my future might contain only a very limited set of dreams, ones that had to be modified to account for my chronic illness. I could not let this happen.

By Day Four I'd passed through the darkness that was clouding my vision. On the other side of all the pain and discomfort was a physical result I could really feel within every fiber of my being. Feeling as if all of the poisons had now been expelled from my system, my body and mind were clear. I'd emerged from the tough first days and the sun was starting to shine. Now all I had left was another fifty-six days!!!

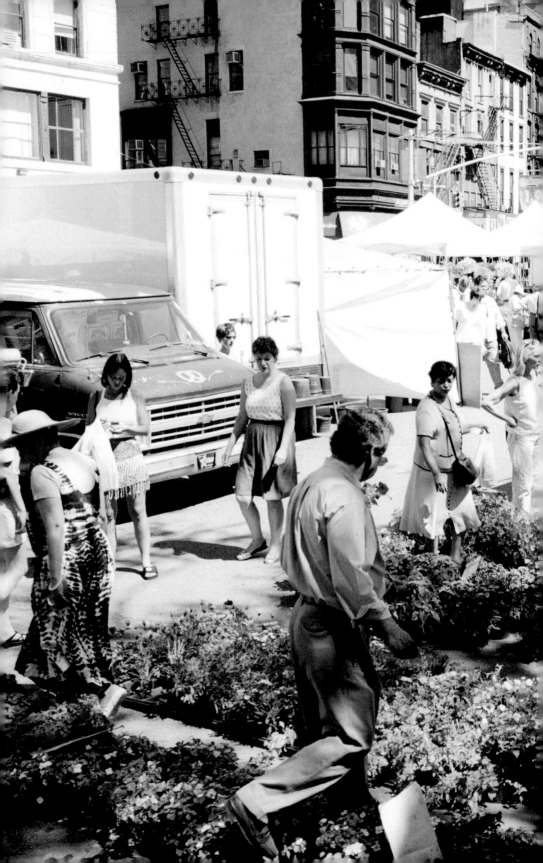

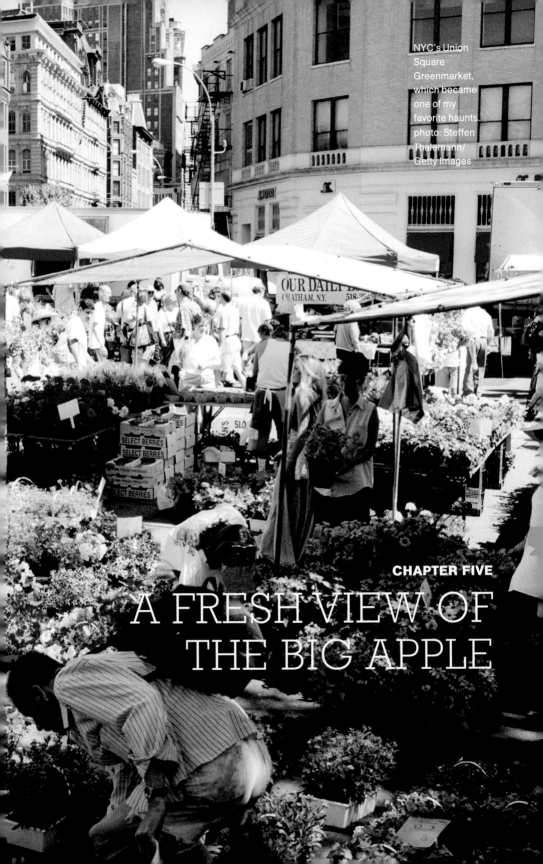

NYC's Union Square Greenmarket, which became one of my favorite haunts. photo: Steffen Thalemann/ Getty Images

CHAPTER FIVE

# A FRESH VIEW OF THE BIG APPLE

I INDULGED IN MORE THAN
A LITTLE WINDOW-SHOPPING
IN NEW YORK CITY, THE HOME
OF THE HAMBURGER AND THE
HEART OF PIZZA COUNTRY
(SORRY, CHICAGO).

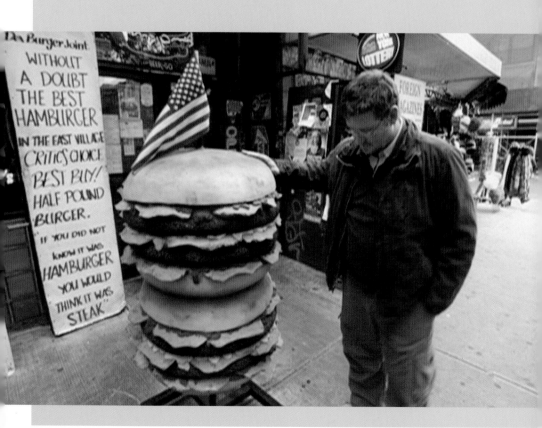

I've always considered New York to be one of the greatest cities of the world. From the Financial District and Lower East Side to the Upper West Side and Harlem; the buzz of power, creativity, and possibility is palpable. As a businessman, I've ventured there many times for many reasons: to work, to play...to eat. I could write a book entitled *Eat, Play, Work* dedicated entirely to the island of Manhattan, which has afforded me all three in giddy abundance. But I think my favorite thing about New York has always been the food. Oh, how I loved to eat in Manhattan's finest sushi restaurants and two-bit pizza joints, sometimes twice in the same day. And so it was with great trepidation that we returned to the Big Apple after spending ten days sequestered on Long Island, far from my biggest food demons (not that the Hamptons doesn't have its share of temptations). But now I also had a different kind of fire in my belly, not one of the hunger sort. I was revisiting NYC and challenging myself to discover a new way of *being* there, as in *being healthy*.

The smells seeping from the bagel, empanada, and falafel shops, and the swishing, clanging sounds of happy hour cocktails were still seductive, of course. Smoke, on which rose scents of hot dogs and roasted almonds, billowed from the carts of street vendors. But never mind. I had my juice. Okay, I won't lie. It was hard to window shop and not buy a cupcake or six at the Magnolia Bakery. Nevertheless, I was neither hungry nor really all that tempted. A curious thing happened when I revisited New York. I began to see a completely different side of it, one that had nothing to do with eating, playing, or working.

I was able to reconcile myself to this vastly different way of inhabiting New York by setting out across the city in search of the best juice bars and farmers' markets. I stumbled on nooks and crannies of the city I'd never noticed before, and had a couple of big "Eureka!" moments about places I hadn't previously paid a lot of attention to, like the Greenmarket in Union Square, off 14th St. That place is amazing. To my astonishment, I found it offers about 1,000 different varieties of fruits and vegetables grown by local farmers. Turns out, the place attracts about a quarter of a million visitors each week, and chefs from many of New Yorks best restaurants—including Momofuku, Butter, Union Square

Café, Koi, and Angelica Kitchen—create their menus from what they find there.

Right around the corner on 16th St., I discovered a great juice bar where I often stopped to order a fresh apple juice or what I call a "Mean Green," which consists of kale, apple, ginger, carrot, celery, and lemon. During the course of my Reboot, this was my staple.

I became familiar with a number of health food stores and organics retailers. I also learned a lot about the fruits and vegetables in my juice, like, for example, celery, which is high in magnesium and nourishes the nervous system. Tomatoes are rich in potassium, which is shown to help lower blood pressure, and are full of the antioxidant lycopene, which has the potential to lower the risk of prostate cancer, for one. Kale is the vegetable that offers the most bang for your buck in terms of pure nutrients: it's super-rich in vitamins A, C, and E, all of which support immune function. Cucumbers and their phytosterols can help lower cholesterol, while carrots can contribute to the slowing of age-related eye problems like macular degeneration and offer cancer-fighting antioxidants. Lime juice is high in potassium and calcium, and pineapple is high in the enzyme bromelain, an anti-inflammatory nutrient. Apples are delicious and promote intestinal activity, while protecting "good" HDL

WHAT GOES INTO MY
RECIPE FOR "MEAN GREEN"?

6 LEAVES KALE
1 CUCUMBER
4 STALKS CELERY
2 GREEN APPLES
½ LEMON
1 PIECE GINGER

The whole idea of eating three meals a day, for example...*says who?* Who had made it mandatory that we eat "three square meals" a day, or else?

cholesterol levels in the blood. How much of this can be said of french fries or hamburgers?

At this point I was two weeks into my Reboot. My thought processes were clearer than ever before.

As much as I'd struggled with the Reboot at the beginning, now I was feeling great and loving the effects it was having on me. As I began to relax and really get into it, I had some fun pondering food myths I had always taken for granted. The whole idea of eating three times a day, for example...*says who?* Who had made it mandatory that we eat "three square meals" a day, or else?

It just so happens that the three-meal-a-day custom is really a modern idea for rich, industrialized countries. Most able-bodied Africans and Asians today eat only one main meal a day. Prior to the emergence of the three-meal-a-day ritual in sixteenth century Europe, around the time of the reign of England's Queen Elizabeth, most people ate only one meal a day, two at the most. For more than a thousand years the one-meal system was the rule, and that one meal, which occurred toward the evening, was considered the reward for the arduous labors of the day. It is well documented that the Greeks and Romans ate only one meal a day at the height of their power, and Herodotus wrote that the invading Persians only consumed one meal in the course of the day as well. Some speculate that as those cultures got richer and more powerful, they began to indulge in eating a lot more, and this over-consumption might have had a hand in leading to their eventual declines.

It eventually became more common, at least in the Western world, for people to eat two meals a day, breakfast and supper. There's an English proverb from the sixteenth century that says: "To rise at six, dine at ten, sup at six, and go to bed at then, makes a man live ten times ten." But as England became more industrialized and prosperous, people increasingly began to eat three meals a day, more as a convention reflecting social status than as something necessary from a nutritional or physiological point of view.

Anyway, long, ponderous walks in Central Park will do that to you, and I liked the idea that my Reboot was prompting me to ask questions

Here I am preparing to celebrate Halloween dressed as Elvis. My costume is still a bit tight, as you can see.

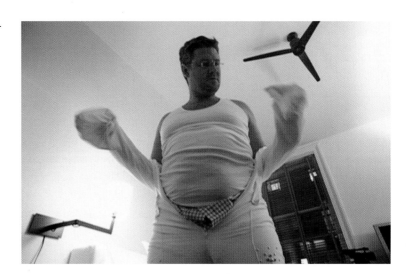

about our most basic assumptions. What I loved even more was the sense of clarity and my vastly increased level of energy. Optimism was oozing from me and I didn't feel at all tired or lethargic. I was making sure to stay hydrated, drinking lots of water, which also helped me to control many of the food cravings I was having. I purposely said "cravings" and not "hunger." I was getting the nutrition I needed and filling my stomach with juice and water, but that didn't mean I didn't crave the things I wasn't indulging in anymore.

Soon enough, I needed to find ways of releasing all that extra energy the Reboot was producing in me. That meant I felt like exercising, and I went on even more long walks around the city. The hunger had left me, and yet my taste buds were coming to life in appreciation of the natural flavors in the various fruits and vegetables I was ingesting through my juice. I indulged in more than a little window-shopping in New York City, the home of the hamburger and the heart of pizza country (sorry, Chicago). I even sauntered into a pizza parlor on Astor Place in downtown Manhattan and inhaled, thinking: *Just two weeks ago, I would have had two of those, and I'm not talking about two slices—I'm talking about two entire pies!* That smell of pizzas baking in the oven is almost irresistible, but walking back out into the crisp autumn air, I felt somehow satisfied with just taking a long whiff.

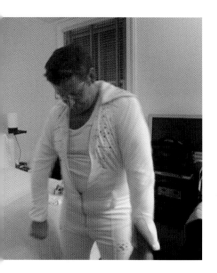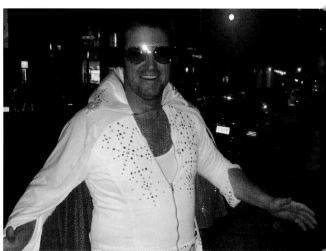

By Day Twenty-One, still under Dr. Fuhrman's observation, I had lost nearly fifty pounds and was down to 7.5 mg of Prednisone. Halloween was upon us and I vowed to get into the New York Halloween spirit by marching in the annual parade through Greenwich Village, which is typically pretty outrageous. I'd never been one of those people who dress up on Halloween, but this year, I decided to suit up as one of my favorite American icons, Elvis Presley.

Although I'd lost a nice chunk of change around the midsection, my body still resembled the King's during his Las Vegas period. So that's the look I went for: an unforgiving, tight, white jumpsuit. The costume was more than a little snug, but I felt confident that the following year I'd be rocking the early-Elvis, Jailhouse Rock look.

After the parade, I wandered through Washington Square Park and marveled at the natural exuberance of the NYU students and others who set out wearing angel's wings and all manner of wigs and costumes. I had to admit, I felt as energetic and full of possibility as they looked. I wanted to tell them to do whatever they could to retain that feeling forever, maybe even saving a specimen of it for those dark days when it will feel like their bodies are rebelling against them. I even wanted to say: "And if that fails, kids, Uncle Joe's got the Mean Green for you right here!" This being Washington Square Park, and me being a middle-aged foreigner in an Elvis suit, I didn't say as much for fear of getting arrested. Instead I sat, watched, and wondered, *When did I stop feeling so young and energetic? Why?* I knew now that things didn't have to stay that way.

We all die eventually. Our brittle, elderly bones might break, we could have great difficulty getting around or end up bed-ridden; maybe we'll suffer from dementia or an assortment of other syndromes associated with old age. Such is life. But must sickness be a *given?*

I couldn't help reflecting on the life of the man whose likeness I inhabited for the night. Elvis was fat and sick like me and died at forty-two, around the same age I was that Halloween. He'd reconciled himself to living a life dependent on pharmaceutical medications because he could think of no other way to cope with the ailments of his body and soul. He died before his time, but he was also quite simply *living before his time.* In the 1970's, the prescription drug was still a bit of an anomaly.

Now in the new millennium, we live in a culture where it's commonplace to dispense drugs like they're candy. New drugs are always being created and marketed to counter the effects of our self-destructive eating and lifestyle habits. The problem is that our bodies always pay a price for taking these medications. They may have toxic side effects that may be known, or are yet to be determined. Further, these medications don't usually cure. Instead, they serve as enablers, permitting us to continue our bad habits while lessening or controlling the effects of those behaviors.

I'm by no means blaming America for this because I admire her and her people too much. It's become a global social disease, in any case. Sitting on that bench in Washington Square Park, I thought about Elvis and I thought about New York and I thought about America. My Reboot was well underway, aided in no small part by all that was available to me in this vast city. But what about the rest of America? I thought about the lyrics to an old Simon and Garfunkel song, "America." Paul Simon and Art Garfunkel were songbirds who had once hung out in Washington Square Park. With my juicer in tow, I was determined to "look for America."

The time had come for me to get this show on the road.

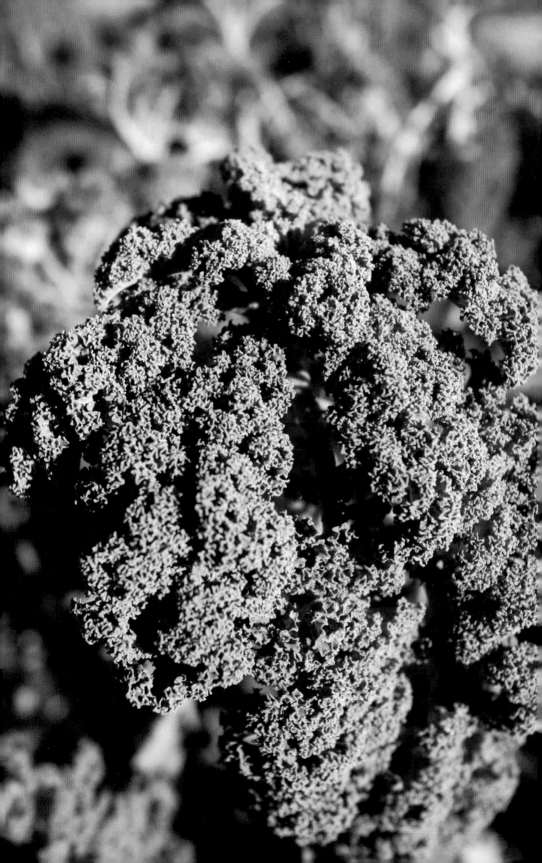

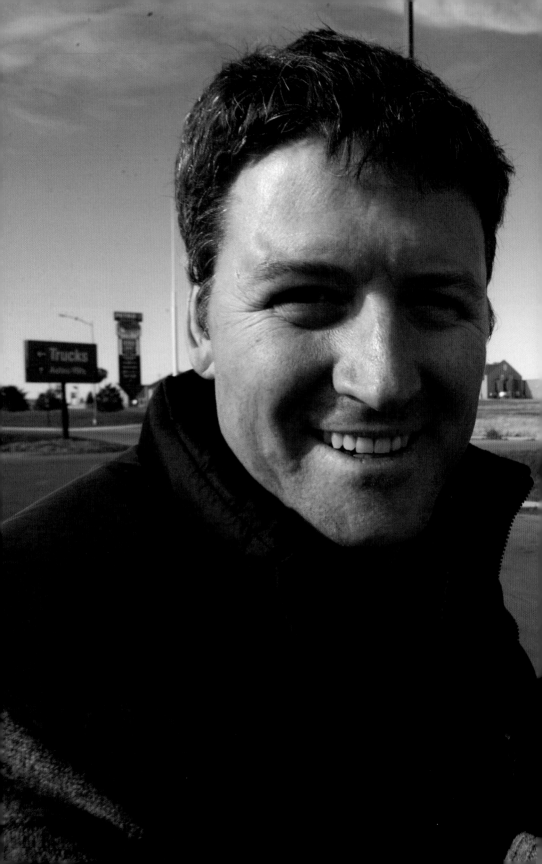

CHAPTER SIX

# MY GREAT
# AMERICAN
# ROAD TRIP

GOING ON A ROAD TRIP WOULD GIVE ME MORE TO DO AND BE A DISTRACTION FROM THE FACT THAT I HAD NOT EATEN ANYTHING SOLID FOR THIRTY-ONE DAYS.

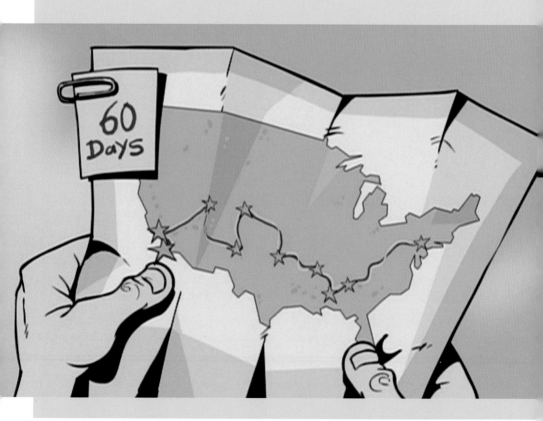

On the morning of Day Thirty-One, I was only too aware that I was at the halfway point of my Reboot. Believe me, when you're drinking nothing but juice and water for sixty days reaching a halfway point is cause for celebration. One down, one to go, was what I said to myself. From this day forward, I'd have juiced for more days more than the time remaining in the Reboot. On top of that piece of good news, I'd lost fifty pounds and had already reduced my Prednisone dosage to 7.5 mg, and had had no new urticaria outbreaks—a huge accomplishment, which meant that what I'd been hoping would happen, that is, that my body would begin to heal itself, was in fact happening.

I was about to embark on another first in my life, which was another reason to celebrate. I was preparing to drive across the United States of America from coast to coast, something I'd always wanted to do, though, come to think of it, when I'd dreamed of doing it, being on a sixty-day Reboot and bringing a film crew along with me hadn't been part of the fantasy. I had to wonder if anyone EVER had driven across the U.S. under these conditions.

Like any road trip, ours required some preparation. I'd bought a blue Toyota Highlander Hybrid to make the trip. I bought a generator. I threw in my juice extractor and bought an extra-long extension cord. I loaded up the backseat with fruits and vegetables from Whole Foods. Because a film crew was coming along, I rented a fully-outfitted camper van. Among other useful features, it had a sink, which, for the next month would be used frequently when I cleaned my juicer.

On Day Thirty-One of my sixty-day juice Reboot, our two-vehicle caravan left New York for points south. Sitting up front with me was Daniel Marracino, my cameraman. In the backseat were two production assistants and my sound guy, Sergio Reyes-Sheehan. Riding in the van were Karen Pelland, our field producer. A road trip hadn't originally been part of our plan. Initially, we'd decided to fly from city to city, conducting on-the-ground interviews and then heading by plane to the next destination on our list. But ultimately, I decided that driving would be a better option. Going on a road trip would give me more to do and be a distraction from the fact that I had not eaten anything solid for thirty-one days, with

ROAD TRIP
UPDATE:
Washington,
D.C., Day #31
of the Reboot

JOE'S
WEIGHT:
262 lbs
(down 47 lbs!)

JOE'S
PREDNISONE
DOSAGE:
7.5 mg

twenty-nine still left to go. I also thought it would give me more of a chance to really get to know the country, and give the film a more interesting backdrop. So we set off to find out what people around the country were eating, and more importantly, what they weren't. Admittedly, it wouldn't be *Easy Rider* and I was certainly no Dennis Hopper, but then again, the sights and experiences I was aiming for were quite a bit different.

Speaking of movies, making them, as it turns out, is a lot harder than it looks. Before our filmmaking adventure, I was a complete novice. There is nothing like a trial by fire to get a person up to speed quickly. I soon learned why it is so tough to make a good film. There are so many variables, from the unpredictability of the weather, to the reliance on functioning equipment, to whether or not your crew agrees on the vision or gets along with one another. And those are just the basics.

Fortunately, I had a great team working with me, but still, here are just a few of the daily obstacles/challenges/considerations we faced: getting permission to film in all the places we stopped, batteries dying, noisy cars ruining our audio, where and when to feed the crew, parking, malfunctioning microphones, the endless loading and reloading of gear; and finally, personality conflicts and creative differences, such as those that arose when trying to decide where to film and why. We were acutely aware of the fact that, at least on paper, our subject matter wasn't inherently suspenseful or dramatic. What we had was an unhealthy, fat bloke on a Reboot, confessing his past sins to others who were mostly in the same boat. No Shakespearean conflict there. I was also no Michael Moore. It wasn't my goal to take on an industry, company, or government, or to vilify anyone or anything. Really, what we were doing was conducting one big science experiment using me as the guinea pig. At the end of the process, would the film come alive? I hoped it would, but we didn't know for sure.

In theory, most documentarians hope to educate, enlighten, and positively affect the lives of the people watching their films, perhaps even save a few lives. But in my case, it was my own life I was trying to save and myself I was educating. If I ended up being successful in my venture, then I would have something worth sharing, something I would be able to

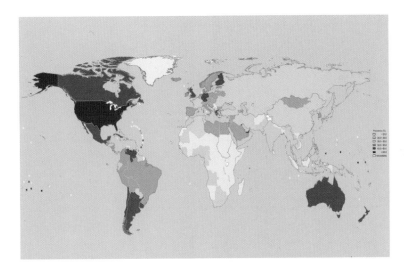

The red areas indicate where obesity is most prevalent in the world—North America and Australia appear to lead the pack!

source: The Centers for Disease Control and Prevention (CDC)

throw out there as a life preserver for others. That goal wasn't even about some sense of nobility or altruism. It's just that I hate wasting precious things, among them, knowledge, which was one of the things I was accumulating by the bucket-load through this experience.

Another thing I was getting very good at was waiting in parking lots for my crew to finish their meals. With six of us on our trip there were five mouths to feed, and I found that it was easier just to stay outside while they devoured diner or restaurant meals of eggs and bacon, cheeseburgers, pizza, Mexican, pasta, or whatever else they wanted. I tried to just wait patiently in the car, sipping my Mean Green, though this didn't mean I wouldn't closely question them to find out what they'd eaten.

Something else I discovered on our road trip/Reboot was that somehow I was no longer finding driving exhausting, as I had on past car trips. I'm pretty sure the reason for this was that I was juicing, which meant that I wasn't stuffing myself with the kind of snacks that give you a little burst of energy at first, and then soon leave you feeling drowsy. Instead of battling sleepiness or feeling tired, I was on fire, alert and full of energy, and taking in all of the sights around me.

That fog I'd felt during the first week in New York had completely lifted and I was on a high. I felt excited about meeting people outside the

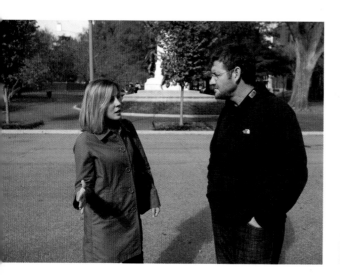
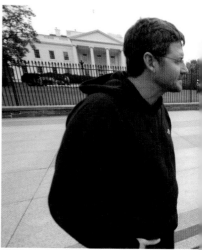

Some of the people-on-the-street interviews I conducted in Washington, D.C.

city. The euphoria I was feeling had to do with surviving the first, detoxifying half of my Reboot and finally reaping its benefits—clarity, energy, and a new sense of optimism. I reflected on something I'd read, that we only normally use about 2% of our brain-power. I reckoned I'd doubled that in that first month! As an added bonus, people had begun commenting on how good I looked and how much weight I had already lost, as well as complimenting my persistence for sticking with it. A couple of weeks before I'd felt as if I'd been walking straight into a hurricane. Now I felt the wind at my back, propelling me forward.

Was I getting hungry? Not really, although my hunter-gatherer instincts were now razor sharp, which meant, among other things, that I could smell a pizza from four hundred yards away, at least. I found that this new trait would stay with me throughout the trip whenever I got within miles of a rest stop or service station where tantalizing pizza slices lay sunning themselves under heating lamps, all greased up and ready to do their bit for heart disease. I was also dreaming about food. I even woke up one morning feeling guilty and very upset with myself. I'd dreamed that I'd broken my Reboot by eating something deliciously awful, like a juicy cheeseburger chased down with a chocolate shake, just like the old days. But then it was back to reality.

The unhealthy eaters all knew and acknowledged that they were committing a form of slow suicide, but that wasn't prompting them to make a change.

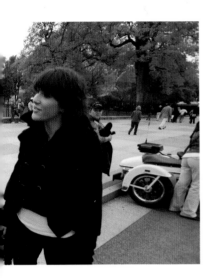 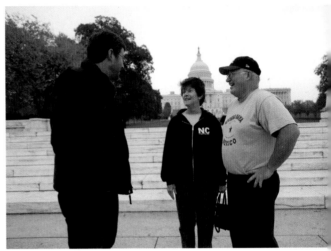

I had made it halfway up the mountain and was seeing things clearly and differently. I could feel the transformation happening within me. Momentous change was also the theme of the moment for the entire country with the 2008 U.S. presidential election in full swing, which was one of the reasons we'd decided that our first stop on the road trip would be Washington, D.C.

Arriving in Washington, D.C., I could immediately feel the electricity in the air, the excitement. I thought about all the marches and protests and other events that had taken place there over the centuries. Right up on Capitol Hill were men and women who'd been elected to office, who had the power to make laws, to change people's lives. I guess if I'd been running for office, it would have been on the fruit and veggie ticket. *"Eat more fruits and vegetables every day—Yes we can!"* I was Rebooting for change.

Among the hot topics of the presidential campaign was the debate over health insurance reform, an issue that was hugely interesting to me, for obvious reasons. But I was curious about one thing: why were none of the candidates, with the exception of Mike Huckabee, who'd himself overcome a weight problem, even mentioning the U.S.'s chronic disease and obesity epidemics when they talked about health? It was really sig-

# LET'S MOVE!

The U.S. is experiencing an obesity epidemic, as are many other countries around the world (including my native Australia), which is one of the reasons I wanted to make the film and write this book.

America's First Lady, Michelle Obama, has become one of the most influential voices out there trying to reverse this trend. Her "Let's Move" campaign has put the spotlight on how we can help get our kids on the right track, to "raise a healthier generation of kids."

The Let's Move website is pretty fantastic. It provides great suggestions on how to eat healthier, on how to be more physically active, and on how to take the lead in our own families and communities on this important issue.

There are a couple of features I particularly love. First, there is mypyramid.gov, which helps users create their own optimum personalized eating plan, taking into account that in terms of calorie and nutritional needs, "one size doesn't fit all." Enter your age, weight, height and current level of exercise, and it recommends a diet plan to help you lose or maintain your current weight, with suggestions for a work-out program.

It also suggests you "vary your veggies" and "focus on fruit." Now that's a recommendation I can say I am taking!

For more information go to:
www.letsmove.gov

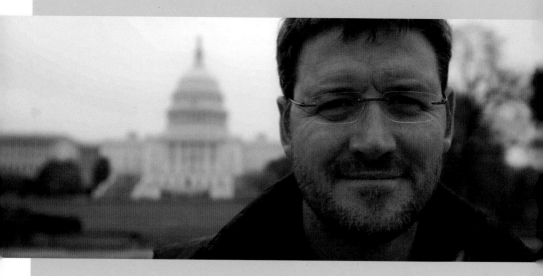

nificant for me to be in Washington at that juncture; in a strange way, I felt like I was there staging my own form of protest—protesting my own addictions—in the very place where so many had come before to change things. I reminded myself, "The ball is in your court."

I walked around the National Mall and continued conducting man (and woman)-on-the-street interviews. I was getting a bit more comfortable in my role in front of the camera by this time, and had learned that introducing my mission to people by sharing photos of myself taken at my fattest, right before I'd started the Reboot, helped set them at ease. My iPhone was getting a workout. The before-and-after shots were real winners because people could see for themselves what a dramatic effect the Reboot was having on me.

There were tourists from all over the country and the world in Washington during my visit, and I was able to talk to a true cross-section of people. I found that once I shared a little of my story, people were often surprisingly open with me about their own eating habits and health issues, especially the women. In general, I found that men were a little less eager to spill the beans. I'd always thought that Americans are generally a very friendly bunch, and now I had my proof.

I was also beginning to observe a pattern, although it was one that didn't surprise me by any means, since I knew that the United States was ground zero in terms of the obesity epidemic, with Australia running a close second. Americans love their fast food. The people I spoke to mostly agreed that they ate it routinely because it was tasty, cheap, and easily available. Like me, they had a lot of rationalizations for their eating habits and were not about to give up their freedom to eat whatever they wanted in exchange for a longer, healthier life without fast food. I was struck, though, by the fact that whatever their explanations, everyone seemed to take responsibility for their own conditions and behavior. The unhealthy eaters all knew and acknowledged that they were committing a form of slow suicide, but that wasn't prompting them to make a change.

Many of the young people I met felt they didn't have to start worrying about what they ate until they got older. They seemed to have no concern whatever that their diets, which were frequently made up exclusively of soda, Taco Bell Chalupas, Big Macs and Whoppers, might be laying the groundwork for future bad health and obesity. This was still a couple of years before First Lady Michele Obama announced her "Let's Move" initiative for addressing obesity in young Americans. But in any case, I wasn't doing what I was doing to judge people or make them feel guilty. Clearly, the stuff we are eating is addictive. The high levels of sugar, fat, and salt that junk food contains are designed to make you want more and more of it. In defense of these fast food-addicted teens, it's not like there is a bounty of other inexpensive choices out there.

In front of the National Museum of Natural History, I met two women in their early twenties who stopped to talk with me about their diets. When I told them what I was doing they seemed receptive to the idea, though this didn't distract them from their mid-morning quest for a hot dog. For me, though, that smoky aroma of hot dogs being grilled by a street vendor had lost some of its appeal, which is one of the benefits of the Reboot. You actually, really do begin to stop craving the foods that aren't good for you and begin appreciating the taste of the simple fruits and vegetables in your daily juice.

Before I left Washington, I made sure to stand in front of the White House and down a juice. Then we got into our cars and headed south.

Our next stop on the Reboot Express was Harrisonburg, Virginia, a historic town established in the late 1700's and located in the beautiful Shenandoah Valley. There, we visited the Downtown Farmers' Market, one of the oldest and best fresh-food markets in the country. To me, it even stacks up to the one in Union Square back in Manhattan. I met up with Marlin and Christine Buckholder, the Mennonite owners of the local, organic Glen Eco Farm. They invited me to tour the farm, and it was an eye-opener.

Besides admiring their operation, I was immediately struck by their commitment to what they were doing. Growing organics involves a lot of intensive manual labor and is a hard climb from a financial point of view, for all kinds of reasons. While it's now changing a bit for the better, government agricultural subsidies still greatly favor big agro-businesses

*The fact that junk food is ever-present doesn't make it easy for those of us who are trying to break our food addictions.*

over small farmers, and many of the tax breaks and other incentives in the food industry go to the meat and dairy businesses. Ever wonder why a salad costs more than a Big Mac? It is because the amount of money being handed out in the form of subsidies to the meat and dairy industries is way out of whack in comparison to what fruit and vegetable growers get. Price-wise, it's just not a fair fight for fruit and vegetable farmers, and it's consumers who end up with the short end of the stick. But since those subsidies began to be put into place sixty or so years ago, heart disease has risen exponentially. If we consumers had to pay unsubsidized prices for meat, we would probably be eating a lot less of it and heart disease might not be America's number one killer.

Government policies have contributed to the increase in obesity, heart disease, cancer, and other health problems because consumers, especially lower-income individuals, just can't afford to buy as many fruits, vegetables, or sustainably raised dairy and meat as would be best for their overall health and nutrition. This was a key issue I hoped to address in my film. Since fruits and vegetables were the basis of my Reboot, which was saving my life, it was only natural that I stick up for them.

From Virginia we again headed south, stopping briefly in Charlotte, North Carolina, then traveling on to Atlanta, Georgia, where I commemorated my long-term, but now defunct love affair with Coca-Cola by visiting the World of Coke Museum. Though I found it strange that there could be an entire museum devoted entirely to a carbonated beverage, it did evoke very fond memories of my childhood in Sydney. From the time I was a little boy Coke had been among my favorite comfort foods, and visiting the museum was like an art lover going into an auction at Sotheby's with blank check in hand. I managed to avoid the temptation to break down and pour myself a cold one, but while the influence of Coca-Cola on my life was over, its influence as one of the most powerful corporations in the world continued to take my breath away.

By the way, we had a lot of fun in Atlanta. Since I grew up in a big city and much of the traveling I've done is to other cities around the world, I felt at home there. I had a friend from New York named Ellie Mae who was living in Atlanta, and she offered to show me around. As Ellie is a bit of a fashionista, she of course suggested we go clothes shopping, which I willingly agreed to, as my clothes had begun to get very loose on me. I can't tell you how exciting it was not to have to shop at one of those stores for "big and tall" men. We swung by a store that carried lots of brands of jeans, and I took quite a few into the dressing room to try them on, no longer knowing what size I wore. I discovered I had gone all the way down from a size 44 to a 38!

What struck me as we continued further south were all the vivid, varied colors along the way: the blues of the mountains, the lush greens, the orange-yellow leaves, the pink sunsets. Some of my favorite moments involved looking around for a place to pull over and make myself a juice. Because we were making a film, we were always looking for picturesque spots, and there were plenty of them. There was something cathartic about the simplicity of finding a roadside farm stand, carefully selecting the ingredients for my meal, and then making myself a juice. No restaurant, no stove, no fuss, just the delicious taste of the fruits and vegetables against the backdrop of a country road or a mountain ridge. The routine made me feel that I was self-sustaining, and there was something liberating about that.

Some say Americans today receive a signal to consume something every seven seconds. I don't know if this is a verifiable fact, but it certainly rings true to me. As I discovered first-hand during my road trip, going for a drive to get away from it all is a very hard thing to do in the United States. Everywhere I drove there were colorful, in-your-face billboards. They are pretty much inescapable. Many of them advertise salty, sugary, fatty foods, and underscore just how many messages there are out there urging people to eat things that aren't good for them.

The fact that junk food is ever-present doesn't make it easy for those of us who are trying to break our food addictions. All you have to do is stop for gas and go inside to pay: you are inevitably assaulted (or tempted) by the sight and smell of grilling hot dogs, freshly baked doughnuts, and, of course, pizza. Sugar, salt, and fat pushers employ food technicians who use their wizardry to ensure you stay addicted via a concoction of additives, colorings, combinations, and other top-secret tricks. They guard

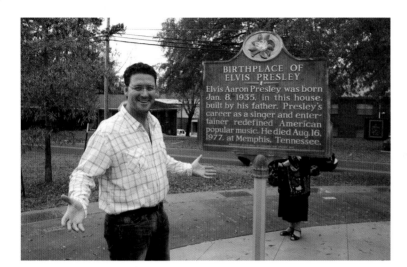

Me, in Tupelo, where the King was born.

their recipes with the same zeal a jeweler guards his diamonds. Just as tobacco executives were finally forced to admit they were putting substances into their products that were purely aimed at creating addicts, I wonder how long it will be before the CEOs of the major food companies have to offer similar confessions. Just remember: when you eat food made by people in white coats, you can eventually expect to be treated by a team of white-coated professionals.

I had put Columbus, Georgia on our itinerary because I'd attended school there for a year as a boy while my father was doing a medical residency. Columbus is located on the Chattahoochee River amid rolling hills and plains, and being there gave me an immediate sense of familiarity.

After checking into the hotel, I got in the car and drove to the place where my family had lived. I walked up and knocked on the front door. The family who now lived there greeted me warmly and invited me in, along with the camera crew. The father of the family had just returned from Iraq. I told them why I was there, and they asked me a few questions and wished me luck. Being there reminded me of when I was just seven years old and receiving my First Holy Communion, an occasion my grandmother, who has since passed away, traveled all the way from Sydney to celebrate with us.

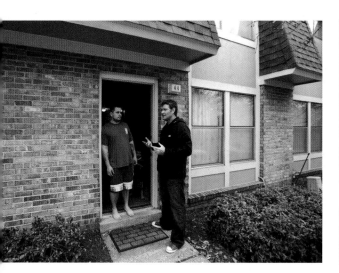 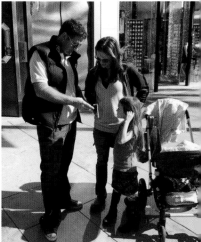

Next, the crew and I went back to my old school hoping to get some film footage, but we weren't able to get in. So we spent the rest of the day exploring the recently revived, historic downtown, and then packed it in for the night.

The following day, we headed further south through Alabama, passing a lot of natural beauty along the way. We stopped at a particularly gorgeous spot alongside a river, where I got out to make myself a late afternoon cocktail of vegetables and juices. Ironically, the spot was right next to a hamburger stand, so I walked over and introduced myself to the owner, who told me that his hamburgers were considered the best in Alabama. He offered me one. I explained that we were actually making a film about a sixty-day juice fast and that I'd pledged to consume only fruit and vegetables for the entire time, so burgers were out. I offered him a juice, and we each toasted to the setting sun. I promised him that if I ever went back to eating hamburgers, I would be sure to look him up.

Did I want a burger? Honestly, not at all by then. It wasn't the burger itself that sparked my imagination: it was the idea of chewing. I was missing the simple act of chewing solid food.

Next stop, Tupelo, Mississippi. Birthplace of Elvis, and host, every June, of the Elvis Presley Festival. I'd also read somewhere that before

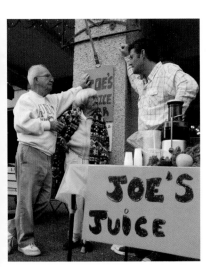

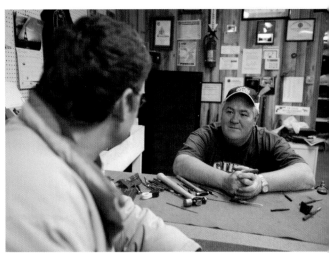

being named Tupelo, the town had been called Gum Pond because of the prevalence of black gum, or tupelo, trees in the area. Interesting, the facts you acquire while on a road trip like ours.

Me, here and there around the country, spreading the word

As for Elvis, like me, he wrestled with junk food and prescription drug dependence. He died fat, sick, and on his throne, which was not the best way for the King to surrender his crown...

While in Tupelo, I set up a roadside juice stand I called Joe's Juice Bar, which looked a lot like those lemonade stands kids set up on hot summer days. But it was November, and it was getting pretty cold. Initially, I wasn't getting a lot of customers, even though I was giving away the juice. But eventually, curiosity got the better of passersby, especially when I started making my own favorite juice combo, Mean Green, which can at first look a little strange to the uninitiated. It is a deep, vivid green color that is quite unlike most other beverages out there. At the same time, it has an earthy appeal that makes people want to try it. We all know we are supposed to eat our greens; one look at a Mean Green and you know that, micro-nutritionally speaking, it possesses radioactive qualities. It literally glows with goodness! I ended up making quite a few converts that day.

From Tupelo, we headed to another musical capital, Memphis,

The local government has, in effect, banned fast food chains from opening in their town, something at least a dozen other U.S. municipalities have

Tennessee, and then on to Guthrie, Oklahoma. It so happens that Guthrie was the original capital of Oklahoma and today is a perfectly preserved enclave of Victorian architecture, a designated National Historical Landmark. With its authentic flavor of the Wild West, it turned out to be a lot of fun for a guy who'd been obsessed with being a cowboy as a kid.

Fittingly, we found our way into a gun shop. Personally, I'm not much of a gun person, but that was one of the reasons I thought it would be interesting to chat with the owner and his wife. They were happy to talk with us. Both were pretty overweight. The owner, Terry, shared with us that he and his family went out to eat most nights, almost exclusively for fast food. He'd recently given up smoking on his doctor's orders, but told us he had no intention of giving up the food he loved to eat. He said he'd rather die "fat and happy."

Fair enough. I knew all about trying to live life as a fat and happy man, but in this regard, I had failed. I'd been fat and miserable. If Terry was lucky, maybe he would end up living a long life and then dying "fat and happy." However, the many illnesses obese people face mean they are more likely to endure a lot of pain and misery before slipping through to the other side at a younger than average age. In fact, Americans can expect to spend the majority of their health care dollars during the last few years of their lives. Only the truly lucky drop dead "fat and happy."

I took another look around the gun shop. For me, it was endlessly fascinating to see guns on sale like candy in a candy store. The right to bear arms allows most U.S. citizens to acquire guns for self-protection. Maybe this is a bit of a stretch, but it occurred to me that vegetables play a similar role, protecting us against invaders who want to hurt us. I examined a 9 millimeter and considered replacing it with a large knuckle of broccoli as a guard against cancer. Or how about arming concerned citizens with a bunch of carrots as protection against cardiovascular disease? Of course, the veggie vigilantes would need a strong lobby group. I could invite the NRA (National Rifle Association) to convert to the NVA (National Vegetable Association), whose singular goal would be to educate Americans about the dangers of heart disease, diabetes, and obesity, and how these things infringe on a citizen's right to life, liberty, and the

also done by adopting zoning laws that prohibit "formula restaurants" like McDonald's, Burger King, and Subway.

pursuit of happiness. I was momentarily tempted to share my vision with the gun shop owner, but he was armed with a 12 gauge while I was just holding a juice!

On to Lindborg, Kansas, which was a place I'd never heard of before we began planning our trip. The town is known as Little Sweden, U.S.A., as it was first settled in the 1800's by a group of Swedish immigrants and is still home to the annual Svensk Hyllingfest, a well-established Swedish cultural festival. It's also where the Anatoly Karpov International School of Chess is located. But for me the most interesting thing about the place, and the reason for our visit, is that there is no fast food to be had within the city limits—none whatsoever. The local government has, in effect, banned fast food chains from opening in their town, something at least a dozen other U.S. municipalities have also done by adopting zoning laws that prohibit "formula restaurants" like McDonald's, Burger King, and Subway. Why? Because they are *health hazards* that have a negative impact on the community.

In Lindborg, I also got my first taste of motivational speaking since embarking on the Reboot. One night, I spoke before a crowd of fifty or so at a local Lutheran church, where I talked about my journey, how it was going, and what had prompted me to do it in the first place. I did pretty well. No one fell asleep and I received a lot of positive feedback afterwards. Yes, here I was, now officially delivering a speech about healthy eating on my fruit and veggie soapbox. I also found out that there were quite a few people in the audience who also had experience with Prednisone. It was a pretty responsive audience, who at the end of my talk flocked to the temporary juice stand I'd set up, where I was serving shot glasses filled with Mean Green. Giving the talk forced me to evaluate and assess what I had learned and how best to go about sharing that information. In Lindborg I found out that there were many other examples across the U.S. where government and people are trying to take back control of their nutritional health.

San Francisco, for example, is the first major American city to forbid restaurants from offering a free toy with meals that contain more than acceptable levels of calories, sugar, and fat. This means that not only has

FACTOID:
Only 22% of Americans get the recommended daily servings of fruits and vegetables. Recommended number of servings: 5. Average American intake: 2.5. And many think the recommended amount is way too low anyway!

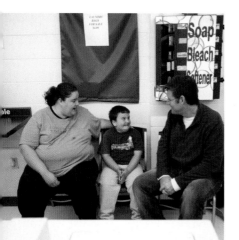
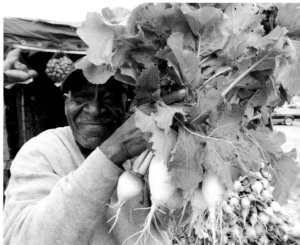

San Francisco's Board of Supervisors voted to ban McDonald's Happy Meals, but they've also required restaurants to provide fruits and vegetables with all meals that are accompanied by toys and served to children.

Now that I was around Day Forty-Five of the Reboot, I was still feeling good. I was continuing to enjoy the increased sense of clarity and the lightness that seemed to go hand-in-hand with juicing, but I was also honestly starting to feel a little anxious: after my sixty days were up, would I have a hard time avoiding foods that were bad for me so that I could completely rid myself of the urticaria and get off Prednisone 100%? That was my next goal. By this point, I was down more than sixty-five pounds and had cut my Prednisone intake from 15 mg. to 3.5. Still, I worried that once I returned to my regular routine and to the rhythms of my life back in Sydney, I would backslide.

One of my perverse pleasures had become asking for a full report of all the meals consumed by the film crew, who didn't seem to mind at all that what they were eating was quite a bit different from what I was ingesting. For instance, I questioned them, did they have bread with the onion soup they ate last night in addition to the cheese croutons? Was the bread whole grain or sourdough? Had anyone ordered the fettuccine? Aha! How was the creamy sauce that accompanied it? As I was

I'm crossing my fingers that somehow the message that you don't have to feel hopeless when it comes to your health will get out there and reach people

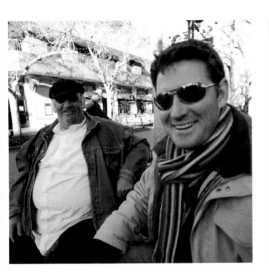
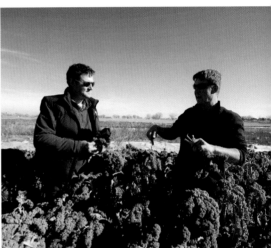

paying for these meals, why not torture myself a bit more with all the gory details? This sort of food voyeurism is something all Rebooters will be able to relate to at one point or another. When the moment arrives—relax and enjoy it!

As much as I was still enjoying the processes of both Rebooting and making a movie, I had also started to feel a little bit like Forrest Gump making his way across the country, telling his story to all who would listen—on park benches, in laundromats, in parking lots, coffee shops, on street corners, in gun shops. I had gone from being a guy who'd spent the last nine or so years trying to conceal the fact that he had a chronic illness, trying to cover up his expanding belly by wearing loose-fitting shirts that resembled tents, to stopping random strangers to tell them about my urticaria and show them pictures of me at my fattest. My grandmother, rest her soul, would have been pleased that that Catholic in me, needing to confess, was finding a lot of listeners.

Soon, we were passing through Boulder, Colorado, a beautiful town with a progressive, health-conscious population and a lot of choices in terms of organic produce and other good foods. There, I met a kale farmer and toured his farm. As we've previously mentioned, kale is high in calcium, iron, fiber, potassium, and Vitamins A, K, B6, and C, as well as

ROAD TRIP
UPDATE:
Lindborg,
Kansas,
Day #45 of
the Reboot

JOE'S
WEIGHT:
244 lbs
(down 65 lbs!)

JOE'S
PREDNISONE
DOSAGE:
3.5 mg

being high in antioxidants. It is a true wonder food. On Dr. Fuhrman's nutrient-density chart, kale is the permanent tournament leader. For the most powerful vegetable on the planet, the process of growing kale is comparatively low-key; it just needs some dirt and a bit of protection from frost. I took a few bunches with me for the road, knowing they just might be the ones that delivered the killer blow to my prednisone dependency.

The most memorable and moving experience in Boulder by far was meeting Dominic Lanza, a man very much down on his luck. We sat together on a bench and exchanged stories about where we were in our respective lives. He was extremely overweight—about 380 pounds, he told me—and pretty much destitute. He confided that his primary diet consisted of pies, cakes, and hamburgers. He considered his situation to be hopeless. As I listened to Dominic's story, I realized how lucky I was to be supported by family, friends, and film crew, and I wondered how I could try and help Dominic, at least in a modest way. I think we established a bond that day and I continue to be in touch with him. I'm still hoping that one of these days something will click inside of him and he'll want to join me in a Reboot to try and get back on track.

# WHY IS KALE CONSIDERED A "SUPERFOOD"?

Until recently I was not a lover of vegetables of any kind, let alone of a vegetable like kale, which is a sort of esoteric vegetable, at least in Australia, where it is still not widely available. But I've come to consider kale one of my go-to veggies for a number of reasons. First, it's got a strong, distinctive taste that packs a wallop and can be used in a variety of ways. It is one of the cornerstones of my favorite juice, my Mean Green.

But the second reason I have become such a huge kale fan is that it is a "superfood" like few others. Kale is a powerhouse that offers an incredible array of health benefits that go well beyond even its incredible nutrient value.

Kale belongs to the Brassica family of vegetables, a category that also includes cabbage, collards, broccoli, and Brussel sprouts. Kale sometimes goes by another name, borecole, which is thought to be Dutch for "farmer's cabbage."

But here is what is really amazing about it: it is rich in anti-oxidants and sulfur-containing phytonutrients. It contains something called glucosinolates and methyl cysteine sulfoxieds, which work to help activate detoxifying enzymes in the liver, which in turn play a role in neutralizing carcinogens. It is filled with vitamins and minerals—A, B6, C, K, calcium, copper, manganese, and potassium, among others. It contains protein and omega 3 fatty acids. Just one cup of it has only 36 calories, but provides 192% of the daily requirement for Vitamin A, and 90% of C (which helps to fight inflammation and oxidize cholesterol—just two of its many benefits).

There have been lots of studies done on this extraordinary vegetable, and it has been found to contribute to:

- Most sustained weight loss ever recorded in a medical study
- lowering cholesterol
- reducing risk of cancer
- slowing loss of mental function
- promoting lung health
- protecting against arthritis
- lowering risk of developing cataracts

How many things in life can you say this about?!

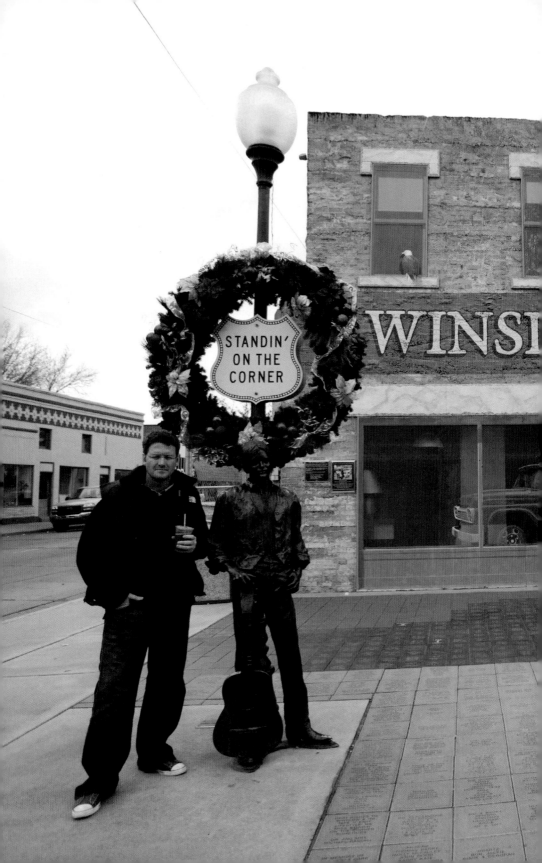

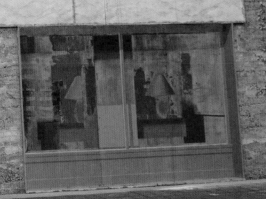

# CHAPTER SEVEN

# FINDING "ME" IN WINSLOW, ARIZONA: FAT CHANCE

I REMEMBER
LOOKING IN THE
MIRROR AND
SEEING A HEALTHY
GUY GOING FOR
THE TITLE OF
"TOTALLY CURED."

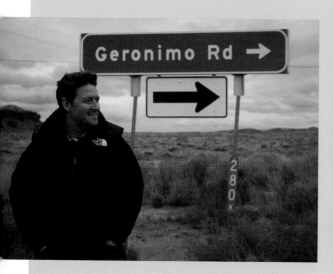
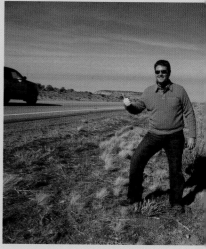

I had almost reached Day Fifty, and found myself becoming increasingly anxious to get to the end of the trip and onto a plane headed back to Sydney. For one thing, it was beginning to get really cold, and I couldn't help thinking of the warm, sunny beaches that awaited me back in Australia. I was still feeling fantastic about what I'd accomplished thus far, specifically, that I'd lost nearly 70 pounds and had been able to reduce my Prednisone intake all the way down to 3.5 mg. But truth be told, I was getting tired of telling my story over and over again with cameras rolling. I was also dying to eat some solid food, which was a good sign: it was my body telling me what it needed. I reminded myself I was only ten days from the finish line and that I was well on my way to healing myself. I remember looking in the mirror on that day and seeing a healthy guy going for the title of "totally cured."

But there was still a lot to look forward to on the road trip. I was excited to get to our next stop of Moab, Utah, which has been immortalized in films ranging from the great John Wayne movie *Geronimo* to Ridley Scott's feminist classic, *Thelma and Louise*. Sergio Leone even set part of the spaghetti western masterpiece *Once Upon a Time in the West* in nearby Monument Valley. And it's pretty obvious when you get there why so many have been inspired by the area, with its wondrous rock formations, spires, ancient Pueblo dwellings, and staggeringly beautiful, red-hued, natural sandstone arches. All I could say was, "Wow."

It's clear at this point that I am starting to come out of my shell.

Moab is situated alongside the Colorado River and is considered the gateway to the Arches and Canyonland National Parks. It is just thirty miles from Dead Horse Point State Park. Moab is also a mountain-bike mecca and an all-round cool town with a pretty health-conscious population. It struck me as one of the most beautiful spots I'd ever seen.

From Moab, we headed about 350 miles south and west to Winslow, Arizona, a stop on the famed Route 66 located in Navajo territory just a short distance from the Painted Desert. The Painted Desert and the adjacent Petrified Forest make up what is known as the Badlands, which extend all the way from the Grand Canyon to make up one of the most scenic sights imaginable.

As music fans know, Winslow was also memorialized in the Glenn

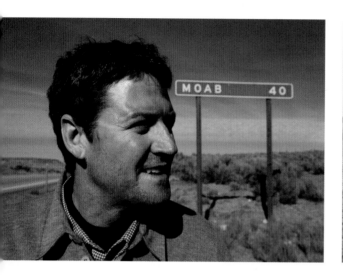

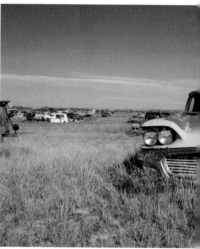

I am thoroughly enjoying our road trip, seeing some of the legendary sights of the American West.

Frey and Jackson Browne classic "Take It Easy," which was named by the Rock and Roll Hall of Fame as one of the 500 songs that shaped rock and roll. Well, we weren't going to be able to take it easy while there, but it was indeed "such a fine sight to see" even though we spent much of our time in a truck stop parking lot instead of taking in the incredible vistas. Ironically, there in that parking lot, we had an encounter that would change the course of our film and have a lasting impact on me.

We'd spent the day trying to wrangle a trucker or two into on-camera interviews with me. The way we reckoned it, if we wanted to talk to people who had some issues with fast food and a sedentary lifestyle, then truck drivers were the Holy Grail. What we hadn't anticipated was that Borat's reputation would precede us. We were conducting our interviews right around the time the movie *Borat* came out. Why was this relevant? Because *Borat's* creator and star, Sacha Baron Cohen, had made it very tough for us to convince potential interviewees that we were sincere. People who might otherwise have opened up on camera were now wary of being taken for fools on the big screen, as some unwitting subjects had after being "interviewed" by the faux Kazakhstani journalist. I was actually a bit flabbergasted by their efficiency in avoiding me, but I found out later that other truckers were radioing their incoming colleagues to warn

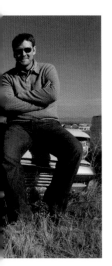
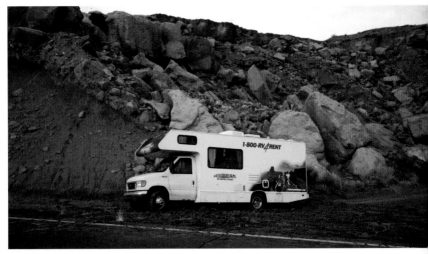

them that there was a crazy Australian armed with a camera who was stalking truck drivers in the truck stop parking lot. All day, we watched as people ran off in the other direction as soon as they saw us coming.

That's when the support vehicle got bogged down in mud...a long day and a whole other story!

By late afternoon, we were cold, tired, and frustrated. I was ready to write off the day as a rare dud. It was about to rain anyway, so I suggested we pack it in and head back to the hotel, but our cameraman, Daniel, convinced me to just wait it out a little longer and at least try to get one or two good interviews in before we called it a day.

I took one more long look around the truck stop and spotted someone sitting in the cab of his truck, which was parked not far from where we stood. I couldn't make out much, except that the guy was wearing a black cap. "He'll do," I thought. I walked over to the truck and tried to get his attention, but like everyone else that day, he was hiding from me. On cue, he ducked down. I banged on his door and rattled off some friendly Aussie banter, as I was by now bored of waiting and had nothing to lose. To my surprise, my confrontational technique appeared to work, as moments later the trucker opened the door and stepped out, slowly lowering himself to the ground.

Now this was done with great care, as the guy turned out to be pretty enormous. Once he stood in front of me, I instantly recognized the tech-

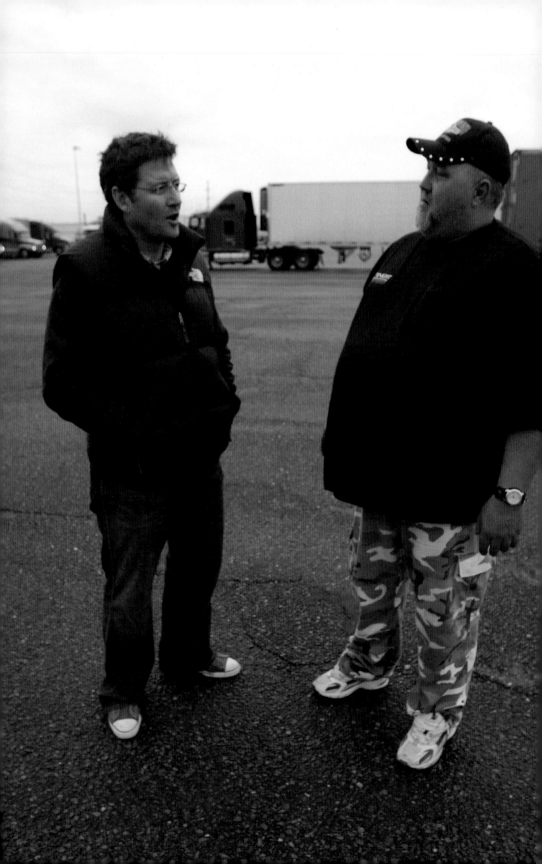

niques of a fat man trying to disguise himself. He was wearing a huge black t-shirt that hung off him like a tent; to shield his chubby, round face, he wore a cap that was pulled down low. As he walked towards the camera crew, I saw that his stomach looked like a huge, round beach ball. He carried himself in a wobbling fashion, as if in pain. Up close, his face was swollen and pasty. His eyes were blue, but the whites were cloudy. He really looked unwell, and it was obvious that he was struggling with his health.

He introduced himself as Phil Staples and proudly announced that he was from Iowa.

By my estimation, Phil weighed at least 400 pounds, which was quite a bit more than I'd ever weighed. I guessed that we were close in age. I explained to Phil what we were doing and why, and then showed him a couple of before and after pictures on my iPhone to drive the point home. Like just about everyone else I'd shared the pictures with, Phil was impressed by the radical change I'd undergone. I told him a little bit more about my mission, my particular illness, and the steroids I was on.

I didn't have to explain much to Phil about the idea of fasting because he, as it turns out, was a pretty religious guy and knew all the stories from the Bible. The concept of a long fast such as my Reboot wasn't particularly outrageous to him. But then he casually mentioned that he, too, had a chronic autoimmune condition that necessitated taking steroids.

When I probed Phil further on this, I discovered that not only did he suffer from urticaria, but that we were both on Prednisone! That knocked my socks off. The type of urticaria I have is extremely rare, and frankly, the last place I'd expected to meet my Urticaria Twin was at a truck stop in Arizona on that cold, rainy day. It was a big moment for me. I'd never before met another person who had my disease. This Phil Staples from Iowa was another bloody me!

The occasion warranted a celebration. I invited Phil to join me for a juice. I wanted to show him how I was healing myself because this was also very relevant to him. I fired up the juicer that was rigged up in the back of my car and made us a Mean Green, comprised of kale, ginger, lemon, carrot, apple, and celery. I could tell Phil liked it, even though it was a long way from his usual fare. As you would imagine, people who drive trucks for

Phil is the "me" I found in Winslow— our meeting changed both our lives.

Phil had become a truck driver because that's what his dad had been...it was the only thing he knew how to do.

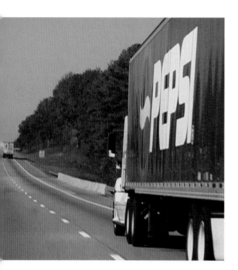
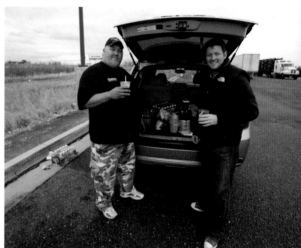

a living are a particularly unhealthy bunch. It's almost impossible for them to find healthy food while out on the road, even if they want to. Truck stops, which are often the only places where they can legally and physically pull their trucks over, serve some of the greasiest, fattiest foods I've ever seen. Truckers also sit for very long periods of time, and have to find ways of staying awake and alert longer than human beings are constructed to do. It's not a recipe for optimal health, to say the least.

All of this was true for Phil Staples. His urticaria, of course, made driving a truck extremely uncomfortable. He confided that his lower torso was prone to blistering due to the pressure from the seat and the effects of the steroids, plus the fact that he spent most of his time sitting meant that his legs and feet were always swollen, particularly his left one. That foot was denied even the minimal workout the right one got operating the clutch and brake. Phil's doctors were concerned that if his condition didn't improve, they might have to amputate his foot. This, along with his massive weight, made it very tough for him to get around.

Phil had become a truck driver because that's what his father had been. He hoped that one day he would be able to stop driving and do something else, but it was the only thing he knew how to do. As a divorced father he had financial responsibilities, though being on the road for

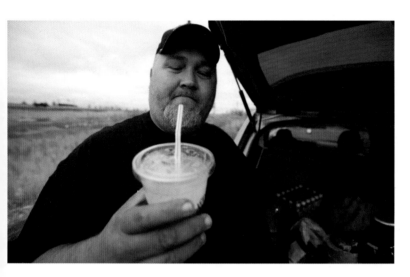

I introduced Phil Staples to his first home-made juice, and he tells me it's not half bad!

twenty-eight days of every month meant that he saw his kids very infrequently. Essentially, his home was the back of his truck, which he shared with a big-screen TV. He told me that being as overweight as he was made him feel ashamed and embarrassed, which meant he kept to himself. The isolation of truck driving was ideal for him in this respect: it pretty much cut him off from having any meaningful contact with the world. On top of everything else, the steroids kept packing on the pounds, a phenomenon I knew all too well.

I felt very bad for Phil. I could see how uncomfortable he was in his own skin, just as I'd been until recently. I asked him about his diet. He confessed that he mainly ate pizza, chips, fried foods, cheeseburgers, candy, and other junk food. Rarely, if ever, did he eat fresh fruits and vegetables. He half-joked: "I'm a hamburger away from a heart attack."

He finished off his juice and I offered him my contact information and a copy of one of Dr. Fuhrman's books, which I thought he might find useful. I told him that if he needed support or advice on how to Reboot his system, he could count me in. I meant it. I felt I already had proof that what I was doing had worked for me, and believed it could also help him to tackle his disease and bring his weight under control. But frankly, I never expected to see or hear from him again.

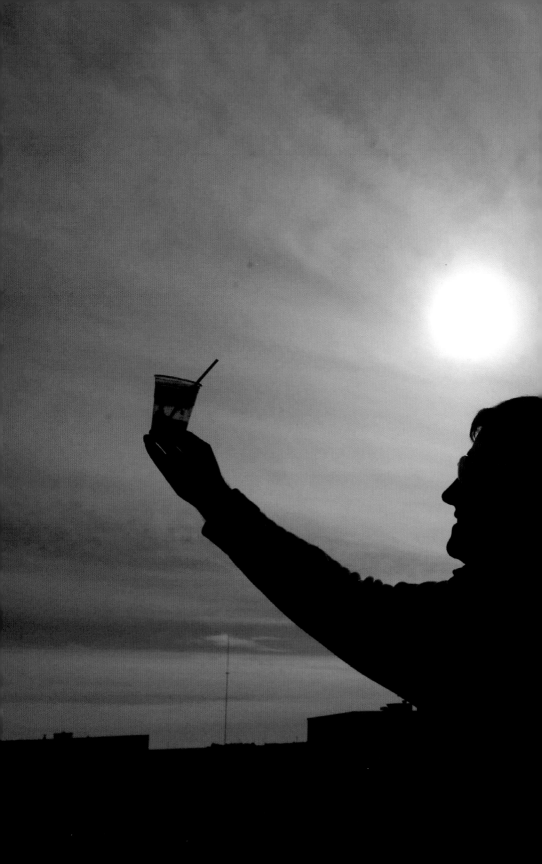

# CHAPTER EIGHT

# HERE COMES
# THE SUN

# SO, HOW DOES A MAN CELEBRATE HIS RETURN TO EATING SOLID FOOD?

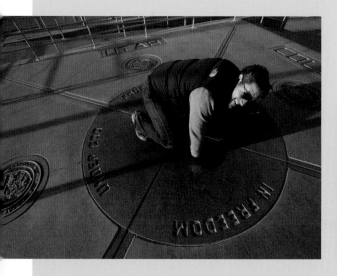

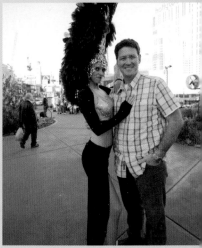

We were back in the car, heading west across the vast deserts and highways of Nevada and nearing the border of California. The air was becoming noticeably warmer, and I was feeling quite a bit lighter in more ways than one. I'd now lost close to seventy pounds, and had nearly weaned myself off the Prednisone – I was down to 3 mg. without a single new outbreak of urticaria. Moreover, my state of mind was nothing short of phenomenal. The sun radiated against a brilliant blue backdrop as I drove, the sort of optimistic sky that only exists in the farthest reaches of the American West. I welcomed the warmth and the optimism as I prepared for the final day of my Reboot. I'd been doing it for so long that I didn't quite know how to say goodbye.

My next destination was San Diego, where the plan was to play eighteen holes of golf on the same course that had been the scene of my health disaster nine years before. After that and another adventure I had up my sleeve, I'd rejoin the human race and start eating again.

So how does a man celebrate his return to eating solid food? Where should he take that first bite of his humble apple (a very healthy way to start the digestive system again after two months of consuming exclusively liquids)? I wanted to reward myself and my crew with something that would be memorable and special. I figured that a ride in a hot air balloon above the Mojave Desert would tick all the boxes. I could defy gravity, stick my head in the clouds, and rise above it all in every sense. It was the perfect symbol for the way I felt, and besides, it would be an opportunity for me to thank the sun personally for growing the food that had saved my life.

That balloon ride, I decided, would be my final adventure before returning to earth and commencing Stage Two of my Reboot, made up of a strict, micronutrient-eating plan I'd pair with regular exercise. Alcohol was also still taboo, and that would be how I'd live my life until I'd completely cured myself, meaning no Prednisone, no urticaria, and a healthy and happy me with many innings of life ahead. I was down more than seventy pounds, and had gotten the Prednisone dosage down to 2.5 mg.

I arrived at the Four Seasons Hotel in San Diego in late afternoon, where, in many ways, I had begun my Reboot journey all the way back

I've almost made it to sixty days, so as a bonus, I am greeted in Las Vegas by a show girl.

ROAD TRIP
UPDATE:
Las Vegas,
Nevada,
Day #52 of
the Reboot

JOE'S
WEIGHT:
237 lbs
(down 72 lbs!)

JOE'S
PREDNISONE
DOSAGE:
3 mg

at the time of my first urticaria outbreak. I checked in, and unpacked for the last time on my road trip. It was certainly good to see the Pacific again, the ocean of my Australian childhood. I indulged in all the requisite clichés: I made the final juice of my Reboot and sipped it on the shore as the sun set. A dolphin leapt out of the sea as if on cue. I was turning every occurrence into something meaningful, so for me that dolphin's gasp of air was an expression of unbounded *joie de vivre,* which I felt by the bucket-load.

I could have spontaneously combusted from the vitality and excitement I felt flowing through my veins. I felt as if I could swim all the way back home to Australia, aiming to arrive at Manly, the beach where I'd spent most of my weekends as a kid immersed in the rough and tumble of the surf. The best part of my days at the beach had always been the ice cream cone I had afterwards, which confirmed that all was good in the world. Such associations between memories and food are deeply ingrained in all of us. Unfortunately for some of us, after we grow up and are left to our own devices, that simple ice cream cone can begin to represent something much more complicated. I had a strong feeling, however, that I would have a new perspective this time around. At the end of the Reboot, I felt I had a far greater understanding of myself. I knew that I would finally be able to moderate my radical consumption habits and find some peace and balance where food was concerned.

I went back to the hotel and got ready for my golf game. I played the eighteen holes, replicating the conditions of my first outbreak of urticaria with the meticulousness of an archaeologist reconstructing an ancient village. On the course, I felt absolutely fine. I had no swelling whatsoever. It felt great to be out in the fresh air and walking again, especially now that I was carrying so much less weight.

My hands did swell up that night, just a little. But in a strange way, I was okay with that. It was a very mild reaction in comparison to what would have occurred two months before, when they would have swelled to the size of boxing gloves with throbbing pain lasting for hours. Now they just tingled slightly. It was interesting for the crew to see what was going on, because until then, my condition had been pretty abstract to them.

You switch yourself off as a consumer, which then enables you to look at life, food, and all the rest of it in a much more objective way.

We didn't dwell on that moment, though. The next day I would get to begin eating solid food again, and for some strange reason, they were more excited about the occasion than I was. Don't get me wrong: I was looking forward to eating. But there was a part of me that was thinking, "I could go another forty days." My body loved the rest I was giving it, and the peace of mind that accompanied the fast was something I would have gladly savored for longer. Being unable to fully enjoy the tranquility a Reboot produces because the whole thing was being recorded was a personal sacrifice I had made. True inner peace is a very rare commodity, so when you go deep into the Reboot process, it is a special gift to enjoy and embrace. Rebooting can put you in a very soulful space that allows you to reflect on the deeper mysteries of the world and your place in it. You switch yourself off as a consumer, which then enables you to look at life, food, and all the rest of it in a much more objective way. In subsequent Reboots, I have allowed myself to really get into that sense of serenity.

Our goal for Day Sixty-One, the next day, was to be in the air by sunrise. My ambition was to see the sun slice through the horizon just as I was biting into my juicy apple. It was still dark on the drive to the launch point and I was thinking about the past, when I'd always bid a fond farewell to my mini-juicing and other health kicks by stuffing myself silly with all the wrong kinds of food, usually enormous quantities of Indian or Chinese. But that was yo-yo Joe, and he was long gone.

I'd stayed on-task and surrendered to my body's natural inclination to be well and healthy. I had to acknowledge that my body is smarter than I will ever be. After millions of years of evolution, the human body has learned a thing or two about intelligently surviving and evolving, especially when our bad habits stay out of the way. My role going forward would be to keep the trend going, infusing my body with optimum micronutrients, encouraging it to heal and Reboot its way back to wellness.

Reflecting on those initial sick and lonely days on Long Island now made me shiver, though I did fondly remember all the people I'd met on the road and the spectacular roads I'd taken. I'd managed to find someplace special to sit down and make myself a juice in every state I passed

That's me, swinging a golf club again for the first time in ages.

That apple sure tasted good!

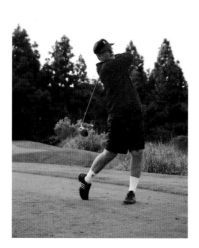

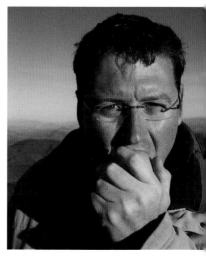

through. All those truck stops, cowboy cafes, laundromats, motels—I knew that I would remember everything about the trip I'd just taken for the rest of my new life. I only hoped that we'd managed to capture the spirit of the voyage I'd taken into myself—and across America—on film, so that I could tell a useful story. It didn't have to be art, but if it wasn't useful or beneficial to others, I would count the whole film experiment as a failure.

When the balloon took off at dawn, I was as excited as I can ever remember being. I was on top of the world, and really, the dawn of a new life stretched before me. My crew, in their own balloon, were as thrilled as I was to finish the project and get home. They had been my witnesses from Day One, and now, here we were on Day Sixty-One. I'd shrunk before their eyes, and they all felt as if they'd witnessed a minor miracle. I have no doubt that at the beginning they'd thought I was mad, but now they could see how healthy and alive I was and how much energy I'd regained. This challenged their preconceived notions about health and how the human body works. They had all become at least part-time juicers, making batches to sustain themselves on long days. Being healthy is infectious. It generates positive energy, and everyone wants a slice of that pie. You will find this out for yourself if you try a Reboot.

When I finally bit into my apple, I must admit that it was something of an anticlimax. Don't get me wrong; it tasted amazing. But my chewing skills were so rusty that I bit—*really* hard—into my cheek! A few more tries and I got my coordination back.

We sailed over vineyards as the sun sparkled on grapes that were destined to be next year's wine—a substance I wouldn't be drinking. It was a bittersweet reminder that Stage Two of my Reboot would require the same level of discipline as the first part. Make no mistake about it; I would have to stick to my micronutrient-eating plan to sustain all that I'd achieved. However, my taste buds were now actually craving micronutrient-rich food; vegetables, fruit, nuts, seeds, and legumes would be my medicine and my treat. I was ready to return to the world of soulful, healthy eating.

For those airborne moments I just let myself think: "Joe—Job well done, mate!" Illuminated by the rising sun, our balloons cast huge shadows over the earth below. I took a good look at that great healer in the sky, our beautiful star. How ironic. Here I was, an Australian who'd traveled to the other side of the globe only to discover that the source of his healing had literally been staring him in the face all his life. *Eat what the sun grows and let no man, woman, or machine mess with its fundamental structure before it ends up on your plate.* That's what being in tune with nature means.

When I'd first conceived of the idea of going on a sixty-day Reboot and making a film at the same time, almost everyone I knew thought I was nuts. I'd thought so too. But after all was said and done, I felt richer now than I'd ever been, and I don't mean financially. During the last two months, I'd gained balance in my mind, which gave me a sense of control. I had discovered the power of nature, with its ability to provide for, protect, and heal all living things, which was something I would continue to harness. I knew I still had a huge task ahead of me—getting down to zero Prednisone by eating well and exercising. I was like a boy pushing a wheelbarrow up a hill—I still had the job in front of me. But now I was more committed to that goal than ever. I didn't ever again want to be afraid to swing a golf club, or to pick up my nieces and nephews in my

ROAD TRIP UPDATE: Aloft in a balloon, Day #61 of the Reboot

JOE'S WEIGHT: 227 lbs (can you believe it?!)

JOE'S PREDNISONE DOSAGE: 2.5 mg

I look triumphant, and I felt that way—even though I knew I still had a lot of work to do.

arms. When I came back down to earth this time, the reign of the boy in the bubble would officially come to an end.

I did something slightly unusual when I arrived back at the airport in Sydney a day or so later. I asked my parents to pick me up, which they hadn't done since I was a teenager. They'd obviously heard all about my adventures and progress, but I knew they were anxious to see what their son would look like walking out of the arrivals gate.

My mother had been very concerned when I'd initially told her I'd be going without food for sixty days. She'd been a nurse, and understood my condition from a strictly traditional point of view involving doctors, hospitals, and Western medicine. How could her boy go to America with a juicer and expect to heal himself? My father, on the other hand, is a physician and also a believer not only in the power of the sun, but in the healing powers of the entire universe. He's studied physics and is a passionate observer of the cosmos. The fact that the knee joint is the most complicated piece of mechanical physics in the human body is why he chose to specialize in orthopedics in the first place. He's also known as a big thinker who believes that if you put your mind to something, anything is possible. He was a bit less surprised than my mom to see his glowingly healthy son stride through the arrivals gate, but nevertheless was thrilled to know that I had at last conquered the diseases of my mind.

My mother couldn't get over how good I looked. I was almost unrecognizable to her. For mothers, I think, a child's sickness has a particularly acute effect. Moms are forever connected to you physically and spiritually, and my obviously renewed health brought her so much joy and relief that she could barely contain herself. Her protective instincts could rest easier knowing that nothing was attacking her son's body anymore.

I saw my brother Tom, who is also a doctor, later in the day. He likened my journey to that of a twelve-step program. While he'd originally been openly skeptical about what I was attempting, he could see that I was a changed man and had overcome my addictions. I was truly honored when he told me he would recommend the Reboot program to his own patients.

I felt fantastic, and I was beyond elated to be back in the Land of Oz. My fitness routine and micronutrient diet could now begin in earnest.

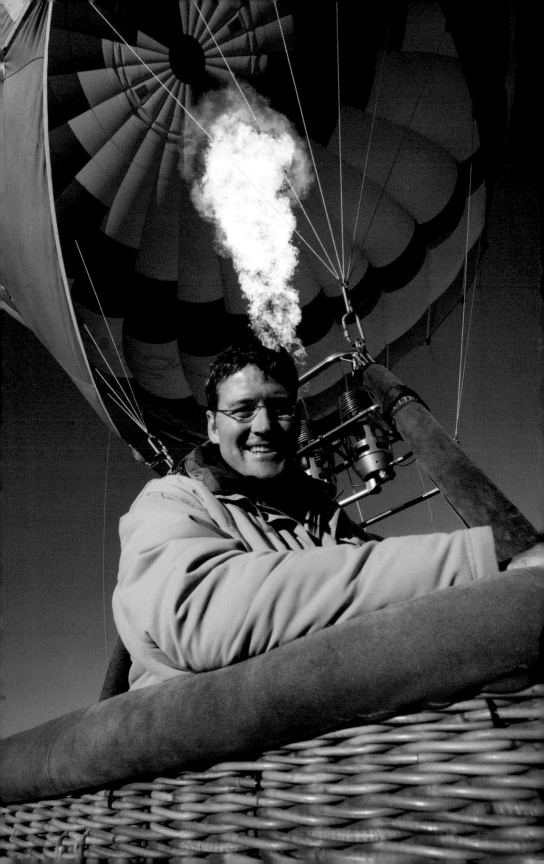

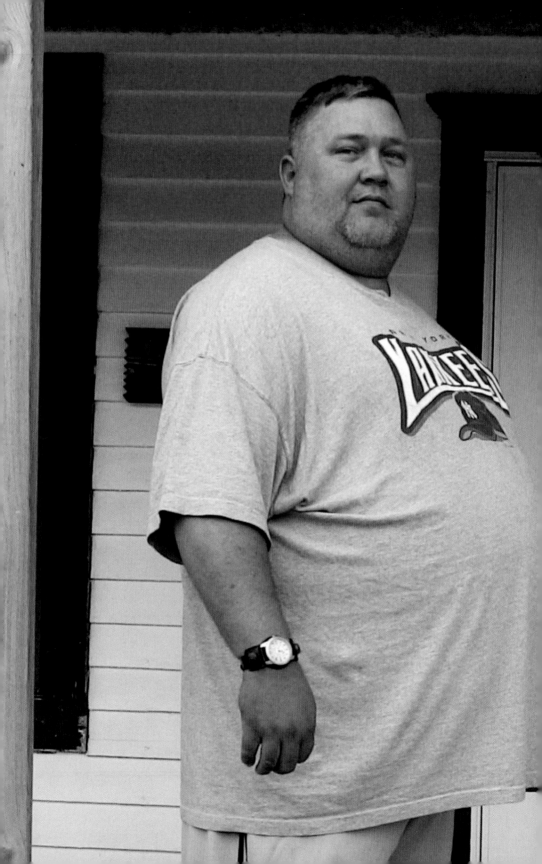

Phil and I,
at the start of
his Reboot

# CHAPTER NINE

# WINSLOW REVISITED

PHIL HAD MADE A HUGE LEAP OF FAITH BY CONTACTING ME, AND WE WERE GOING TO DO EVERYTHING WE COULD TO SUPPORT HIM AS HE GOT HIMSELF BACK ON TRACK.

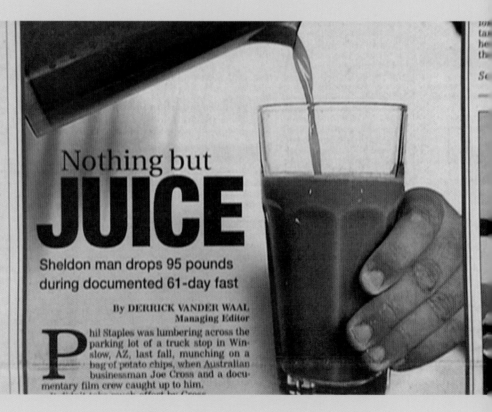

Nothing but

# JUICE

Sheldon man drops 95 pounds during documented 61-day fast

By DERRICK VANDER WAAL
Managing Editor

Phil Staples was lumbering across the parking lot of a truck stop in Winslow, AZ, last fall, munching on a bag of potato chips, when Australian businessman Joe Cross and a documentary film crew caught up to him.

When I was out on the road, I freely gave out my contact information to anyone I thought might benefit from trying a Reboot themselves, which was pretty much everyone I met. I'd been back in Australia for nearly six months, and up to that point, not one person had taken me up on my offer. It takes a lot of guts to stick up your hand and ask for help, so I wasn't too surprised. I've found that the hardest part about reaching out is first admitting that you're in some sort of trouble. Anyway, I was busy enough, mostly celebrating being a normal, healthy guy again. I had continued to eat a micro-nutrient diet from mid-December, when I'd finished the road trip, to the end of February, when I finally became Prednisone-free. I was going for daily morning speed walks on Bondi Beach and regularly lifting weights at the gym in order to build muscle, as well as swimming. Though I'd lost about one hundred pounds, I still had a long way to go in terms of regaining some of the muscle and strength I'd lost in the bad old days.

Things were back in full swing as far as my day job was concerned, and in terms of the social whirl of Sydney. We were doing the post-production work on the film and getting very excited about the great footage we'd shot during my Great American Road Trip.

Newspaper article about Phil's amazing progress and community outreach

When I am on business in the United States, I carry a different cell phone with me than the one I use when I'm home in Australia. When I'm back in Sydney I put the American one away, only checking the voicemail every few days. One day nearly six months after my Reboot, I checked the voicemail on my American cell and was startled to hear the voice of Phil Staples, the truck driver from Iowa I'd met in Winslow. He didn't say much in the message, but I could tell from his tone that something was wrong; frankly, he sounded desperate. What he did say was that he'd decided to turn to me for help because he was running out of options.

I tried calling him back right away, but he didn't pick up, so I left a message. I called him repeatedly over the course of the next few days, but we didn't connect until several days later. What he told me when we spoke worried me a great deal. He said that he felt he was at a crisis point in his life. He told me that his weight was skyrocketing and the urticaria

Phil, on the
first day of our
reunion in Iowa.

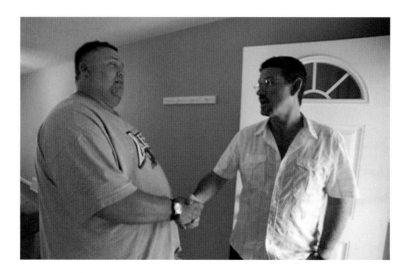

outbreaks were worsening. His state of mind, he confided, was darker
than it had ever been. Now, I didn't know this guy at all, except for our
brief encounter months ago in a truck stop parking lot. But I could identify him in a lot of ways, especially because he and I shared the same rare
autoimmune condition. I had told him way back in Arizona that he could
count on me, and I had no intention of letting him down now. I congratu-
lated him on reaching out for help, and told him I would make good on
my promise.

I got off the phone and thought about our conversation. I was really
worried about the guy. But how could I help him from halfway around the
world? Then it hit me. I would fly back to the United States as soon as I
could manage it and get Phil started on a Reboot of his own. He sounded
ready. I checked back in with Phil and told him what I was thinking. Then
I booked a flight to Iowa.

I had asked Phil if he would agree to let us film his progress and he'd
said yes, so I when returned to the United States a few days later, I gath-
ered up the crew and we set out for Sheldon, Iowa. Phil had made a huge
leap of faith by contacting me and we were going to do everything we
could to support him as he got himself back on track. I'd wanted to bring
him something that would be meaningful and represent a challenge,

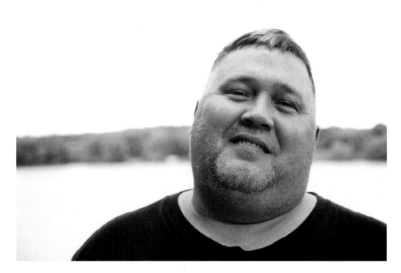

At one time, Phil had been a championship swimmer. Those glory days were long gone, but he was determined to get them back.

so I'd purchased a rugby jersey in the colors of the Australian flag, size 2XL. I guessed that Phil was probably closer to a 5 or 6XL, which was where the challenge would come in: his first goal would be to fit into that shirt.

When I pulled up in front of Phil's house in Sheldon, Iowa, I was feeling better than ever. I'd continued to lose weight and was maintaining a vigorous fitness routine. I'd made good on my commitment to adhere to a micronutrient diet until I was 100% Prednisone-free and hadn't had any outbreaks since the Reboot. All of this made me feel confident that my experiment would also work for Phil.

Phil stepped out of his front door to greet us and I immediately handed him the shirt. He'd gotten even bigger since the last time I'd seen him and was wearing the same kind of oversized, baggy t-shirt as before, which was clearly meant to disguise his bulk. It wasn't working, but I knew from experience what he was going for! He held the rugby shirt up to his chest. Next to him, it looked like a kid's shirt. Phil grinned and said, "I guess that's my goal!"

Another challenge for Phil was that he was in difficult financial straits. His trucking company had refused to allow him to work during the juice Reboot, citing concerns about insurance liability. His current state of

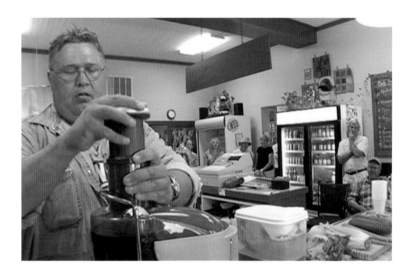

mind had also caused some tension with his employers, resulting in an enforced, temporary hiatus. To make things worse, he'd had to move back in with his parents—not exactly the ideal circumstances for new beginnings. Therefore, we planned something special for Phil's ten-day Reboot: he was going to kick things off at a small, nearby lakeside resort, where I would help him get settled, show him the ropes, and offer moral support. Then it would be up to Phil.

Phil's short-term goal was to begin to feel good enough just to be able to get around more easily, without as much pain and discomfort, and to feel less lethargic and more positive about life. His long-term goal, though, was much more aggressive. As a young kid, he'd been a championship swimmer (I'd seen pictures of him as a budding star athlete, and they presented a stark contrast to Phil now). As a teenager, he'd clearly been a handsome bloke: slim, tall, with a wide smile and long, blonde hair. He wanted to show his children that Phil, the Phil they'd never known: a fit, attractive, still-young man full of possibility.

Before Phil got started, though, it was important to have his health properly assessed and get his doctor's permission to embark on the program. I accompanied him to a local clinic in Sheldon. It had been some time since Phil had had a complete physical, so the first order of business was to get him weighed, which in and of itself turned out to be an ordeal. Phil was too large for the scale they normally used to weigh patients; they would have to use a special scale for him. Understandably, this was very embarrassing to Phil. At more than six feet tall, Phil is a big guy, but his weight told the whole picture: he weighed in at 429 pounds. Next, they took his blood pressure, which, as expected, was high—160 over 84—as was his cholesterol. His body mass index was 58 kg/m2, more than double what was in the desirable range, which is more like 25 kg/m2 (18.5-24.9 is healthy weight). This meant that Phil was considered "extremely morbidly obese." Tests were run on his heart to make sure he didn't have some previously undiagnosed, underlying condition that would rule him out as a candidate for a juice Reboot. Dr. Amy Badberg, a physician who'd treated Phil before and was familiar with his illness, was quite worried about him now. She could see that his health was rapidly deteriorating and talked through the statistics with him, advising him that if he didn't make immediate and dramatic changes in his lifestyle, he would be looking at diabetes, heart disease, cancer, even sudden death from heart failure. Dr. Badberg reiterated her concern about restricted blood flow and the swelling in his left foot, which she advised would require amputation if it got much worse—this was a conversation she'd had with Phil before.

That day, though, she was able to give Phil an all-clear for the Reboot. She thought it was a good idea for him. Before leaving the clinic, Phil scheduled another appointment for the following week. Phil's starting goal: to lose 100 pounds.

Next stop: the grocery store.

One thing that never ceases to amaze me about the United States is that even in regions famous for farming and agriculture, like Iowa, there is often little fresh produce available. But we were able to stock up on fresh fruits and vegetables at the Sheldon branch of the Hy-Vee chain of stores, which carries a wide variety of produce. Phil would be needing a lot of apples, kale, and numerous other items to get started. I shared with him my recipe for making any almost any combo tastier: the addition of lemon and ginger.

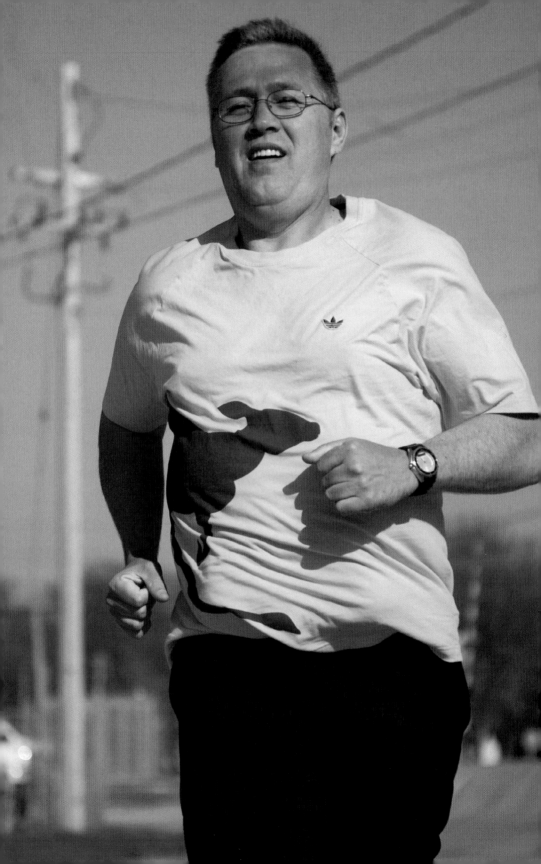

# If no one cares about me, why should I care about myself?

Later that day, I showed Phil how to work the juicer, and the next day he was off to the races making his own concoctions. I also accompanied him on a few short walks to help get him moving.

Incidentally, I'd made a conscious decision not to stay with Phil for the entire ten days of his planned Reboot. I set him up on Day One and then left him to manage on his own, though the film crew was still there to document his experience, albeit under strict instructions not to enable or facilitate. This would be something that he would have to want for himself. I returned to Sydney, but got regular updates from him via cell phone. The first three days of Phil's Reboot were very tough. His body was going through a major detox, which was making him feel incredibly nauseous. He slept a lot and struggled with headaches. He was also still feeling very dark and sad, and shared with us on film some of what was going through his head. He'd begun to feel no one cared for him anymore, and was thinking: "If no one cares about me, why should I care about myself?"

On Day One we had gone for a few walks together, just five minutes out and five back. He gradually walked for longer periods of time. He also went down to the lake on Day Two, slowly dipping his toe into the water and then eventually submerging himself, allowing his body to get used to the feeling of being in water again. He floated for awhile that day, and then got out. Every day after that he went in, each time getting a little bolder.

By the fourth morning of the Reboot, he was starting to feel less exhausted, even starting to have a little energy. In an ideal world Phil's family would have been there to back him up, but his family wasn't yet convinced that the Reboot was a good idea, even though they recognized how badly he needed help of some kind.

After just five days on the Reboot, Phil reported that everything was starting to feel brighter and clearer, and that he was actually starting to feel energetic. He was walking farther and faster, and while he was still getting out of breath, he could feel his endurance building. His appetite was starting to feel satisfied with juice and water alone. Plus, he was swimming, feeling a little rusty still and embarrassed about being in a bathing suit. His stamina was improving stroke by stroke. Once upon a time, he'd been the second best young swimmer in the entire state; now

My gift to Phil, and his challenge and goal, is now something he can wear with pride... and boy, look at him run! When I saw this footage for the first time, I cried.

swimming was proving to be a literal lifesaver, as it allowed him to exercise in a weightless environment.

Everyone at the resort got to know Phil and became interested in his progress. As the pounds came off, he began to come out of his shell little by little. He even began to convince others to try his juice. Remember, good health is infectious!

I spoke with Phil by cell on Day Ten, which was supposed to be the final day of his Reboot, and he told me he'd already lost thirty pounds. He was feeling charged up and wanted to continue for another twenty days. I questioned him to be sure this was what he wanted and that he was onboard for all the right reasons—for himself, and not because of outside pressure from anyone, including me. He assured me he'd thought it through. "I figure I'm down about two bowling balls," he laughed. He was ready to throw down some more. For the rest of his Reboot and even after, he continued to measure his weight loss in bowling balls. As his ten-day Reboot extended into thirty days, I knew that Phil was going for the title that had been my goal, too: "Totally Cured."

I was gratified to see that he was taking responsibility for his own health, and that I'd had the chance to lead by example.

When Phil returned to Dr. Badberg for his first month's check-up, he weighed in at 368 pounds, down 60 pounds from where he'd started. The staff was amazed by his transformation, not only in terms of his outward appearance, but also by the stats. Phil's blood pressure had dropped to 136 over 70, and his triglyceride level had gone from 216 to 161. Even his heart was squeezing more efficiently than before. Dr. Badberg encouraged him to keep it up and indicated that it might be possible for him to reduce or even eliminate the Prednisone if he continued on this path. She gave him the green light to stay on his Reboot for a full sixty days.

To celebrate, Phil brought a container of Mean Green with him to the doctor's office and offered a cup to Dr. Badberg, who was no doubt curious about the healing powers of this mysterious juice. But was it really so surprising that Phil's new medicine was a simple juice? After all, the use of plants and plant substances to cure illness can be traced way back to ancient times.

# RECIPE FOR PHIL'S MEAN GREEN JUICE

(which is different from my own recipe for "Mean Green")

1 BUNCH KALE
4 STALKS CELERY
2 SMALL OR 1 LARGE ZUCCHINI
2 SMALL OR 1 LARGE CUCUMBER
2 GRANNY SMITH APPLES
2-4 CARROTS
½ TO 1 WHOLE LEMON
¼-SIZED PIECE OF GINGER ROOT

Phil gets a little local ink.

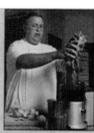

"I wasn't fast enough, so he kind of caught me with his camera crew before I got to my truck," the 43-year-old from Sheldon recalled with a chuckle. "And we talked."

Cross explained to Staples that he was on day 50 of a 60-day juice fast and already had lost about 90 pounds, showing Staples a "before" photo of himself on his iPod. He was juice fasting his way across America — from New York City to Los Angeles — to promote the benefits of the fasting for detoxifying and rebalancing the body. An independent film crew was documenting his journey.

He made up a batch of "mean green" juice

Phil Staples sticks a bunch of kale in a blender as he mixes up a batch of "mean green" juice for his juice fast.

Phil Staples, 43, a longtime Sheldon resident, pours out a glass of "mean green" juice mixed from kale, celery, cucumber, apples, lemon and ginger root. He spent 61 days on a juice fast that saw him lose 95 pounds and drastically reduce his blood pressure.          (Photos by Rylan Howe)

## BEFORE AND AFTER

*It's been wonderful; it really has. The health benefits, the en-*

From Days Thirty to Sixty of Phil's Reboot, he really came into his own. His influence in the Spirit Lake area grew as he shrank and he began to try and convert others to his new cause, assembling a small army of fellow Rebooters who wanted a taste of what he was drinking. He had become a regular customer at The Market, a local health food store. Just as he'd piqued the curiosity of the other guests at the lake resort with his transformation, the staff and customers at The Market who witnessed the dramatic changes Phil was undergoing also became intrigued. The fact that Phil was a fellow Iowan and a truck driver, no less, further heightened their interest. The local newspaper ran a story on Phil, and the "Community Juice Fasting Program" was launched. I got the juicer company Breville to send some juicers to The Market for the locals to use, and a group of customers signed up to do a five-day Reboot. The owner of the resort where Phil had kicked off his Reboot was among those who signed up, as was the wife of a local doctor. One Rebooter who shared a particular kinship with Phil was a bloke named Eugene, also a truck driver. Eugene lost twenty-two pounds in those five days, along with his desire to eat junk food.

Seeing Phil lead that group was an extraordinary thing. Knowing that the man now inspiring others to get healthy had himself been in such

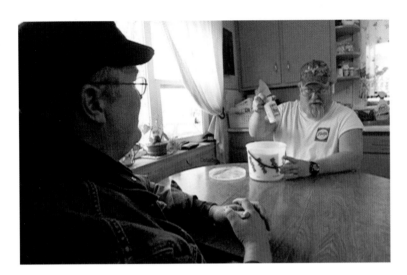

Phil with his brother, "Bear," and his bucket of meds.

desperate circumstances a short time ago was very moving to me. It was another piece of evidence that good health is infectious. Store manager Tammy Hamlin rallied the entire town that summer and four additional Reboots were launched, with equally impressive results. After Dr. Tim Taylor saw the benefits of the Reboot firsthand in his wife's improved health, he began encouraging patients from his practice to participate.

After sixty days on the Reboot, Phil weighed in 96 pounds lighter than when he'd begun. He decided to give up truck driving and got a job at the YMCA in Spirit Lake. He's continued his healthy lifestyle, exercising and eating micronutrient-rich food to get down to around 200 pounds. He no longer takes steroids, and has significantly reduced his other medications. He hasn't had an urticaria outbreak in some time. That Aussie rugby shirt? It actually fits him just right.

I was glad that Phil had joined me in my experiment, confirming what can be achieved by eating only micronutrient-rich food. The Reboot turned Phil's life on its head. While there will always be bumps in the road for him, as there are for me, he now knows that he has all the tools he needs to be healthy, for himself and for his kids.

During the course of Phil's Reboot, I had the pleasure of meeting his brother Barry, who, appropriately enough, goes by the name of Bear.

134

FACTOID:
Painful,
chronic condi-
tions such as
constipation,
irritable
bowel
syndrome,
migraines,
chronic
fatigue syn-
drome, and
fybromyalgia,
aomong many
others may be
alleviated
through
adopting a
plant-based,
micro-nutri-
ent-rich diet.

When I first met him I saw that while he was not as heavy as his brother, he was still obese—up around 340 pounds. He was taking all kinds of prescription medications for a range of ailments and conditions. When we later asked him to show us all his prescription bottles, there were so many that he had to bring them out in a laundry basket. Bear also hadn't been near a fruit or vegetable in quite some time.

Bear admired what Phil was doing, but wasn't ready to try something so "radical." In fact, he told me he really thought the Reboot was just a passing fad, that it wouldn't ultimately help Phil. He was glad his brother was trying something—*anything*—to lose weight, but he was by no means a believer. Then he watched in growing astonishment as Phil lost more and more weight, grew more energetic, and began working out. His astonishment turned to admiration. Still, it took something drastic to finally convince Bear that maybe he also needed to give the Reboot a try.

Looking back at himself at that time, Bear now admits he was "a train wreck." In addition to his weight problem, he was also smoking a pack and a half of cigarettes a day. His diet was awful. Because of his weight, he was having knee problems. One day he went to the hospital for minor knee surgery; the next, he was heading back to the hospital in a medivac helicopter. He'd had a heart attack. It took three stents and several days in the hospital before he was able to return home.

Understandably, the heart attack really rattled Bear, as well as his family and friends. He knew he had to make some big changes. He turned to Phil for help. Due to his diabetes and his heart condition he couldn't go on a full-out Reboot, but he was able to begin a modified version consisting of micronutrient food. He slowly introduced juicing into his daily menu. Together, he and Phil shopped for a juicer, and then for the fruits and vegetables that would become the staples of his diet going forward. Gradually, he was able to rely more and more on juice, and he actually began to like it. He started to lose weight and to feel better, thanks in large part to the encouragement he received from his wife, Claudia, and their daughter, Vanessa. As soon as he was able to, he started some moderate exercise, often with Phil by his side. He began to really develop a taste for the flavor of the micronutrient foods he was eating, and to feel the benefits of his healthier lifestyle. He felt more energetic, which in turn led him to begin exercising more vigorously. His health improved to the point where his doctor allowed him to move to a diet consisting mainly of juice and raw fruits and vegetables. Within fifty days he'd lost forty pounds. Soon he began going to the local pool twice a day to do laps. He was able to go off some of his medications, including the one for diabetes. At the time of this writing, Bear is still working in on his goal of losing 100 pounds.

"People on the east and west coasts have more of an awareness about healthy eating, and they also have more opportunities to eat healthy," Bear told me. "Here in the Midwest," he said, "we can show you 4,300 ways to cook beef. All the fattening food is right here. We literally have to go to another town to find healthy food to eat, which why, I think, it's so easy to get heavy out here in the Midwest." It's not that Bear was trying to relieve himself of the responsibility for his condition. He told me, "It was my mind-set I had to change." This is a task he is working on each and every day.

CHAPTER TEN

# THERE IS NOTHING NEW UNDER THE SUN

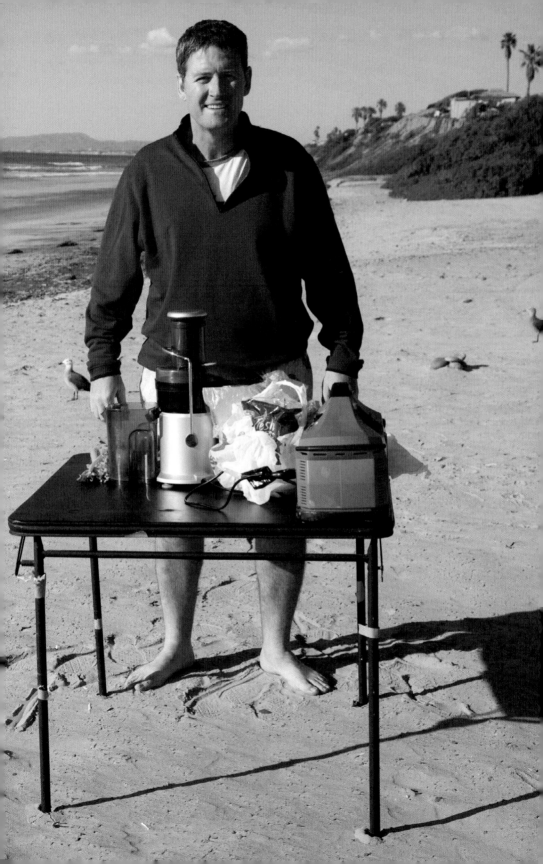

MOST OF THE TIME
WE UNDERSTAND
THAT WE HAVE TO
RESPECT THE LAWS
OF NATURE.

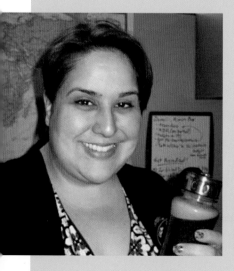
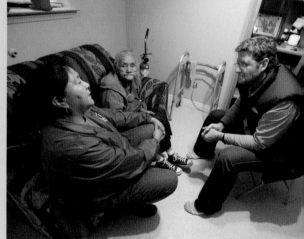

A year or so after I completed my sixty-day Reboot, I travelled to Egypt. I'd never been there before, and I very much wanted to see the ancient pyramids. They date all the way back to 3,500 B.C. and were built by the Egyptians as tombs, as a means of helping usher their kings and pharaohs into the afterlife. The ancient Egyptians knew the power of the sun, which they worshipped. When I think about this, it makes me realize that since humans began to inhabit the planet, all civilizations have recognized the incredible power of Mother Nature. Whether we are talking about natural catastrophes, such as earthquakes and massive storms, or about the laws of physics and science that regulate how long we remain on this planet and in what way, Mother Nature's word is the bottom line.

So the thing is, most of the time we understand that we have to respect the laws of nature. For example, jumping out the window of a twenty-story building without a parachute would not be a good idea, unless we wanted to die. We know that due to the law of gravity, jumping from that window would mean falling straight to the ground. But somehow, when it comes to something as basic as what eat, we often think we can somehow trick nature. We routinely eat and drink and otherwise ingest things that are bad for us and expect somehow to escape the inevitable consequences of our behavior. If we are phenomenally lucky, perhaps those negative consequences won't manifest themselves until we are well into adulthood, when our metabolisms have slowed and our bad habits start to catch up with us. Every now and then, a person may even get off scot-free. But for the large majority of us, we will end up paying the price.

Folks I have encountered along the way.

As humans, we are programmed to respond or react quickly to things that immediately threaten us. For example, if a saber-toothed tiger jumped out in front of you during your morning walk, you could count on the fact that the hair on the back of your neck would stand up, you would feel fear and anxiety, and you would run for your life. So why is it that we are not as concerned about things we know will eventually have a definite negative impact on our lives, such as smoking, drinking alcohol and caffeine to excess, and eating foods that we know are unhealthy? Unfortunately, it seems we don't have an internal mechanism that automatically steers us away from things that will harm or kill us slowly, at least not in the same way that the fight-or-flight instinct prompts us to run away from that saber-toothed tiger. The reason for this is that those instincts are survival tools that have been passed down through evolution over hundreds of thousands of years...tens of thousands of generations. It's only in the past hundred years or so that through ingenious techniques we have developed the means to create the kinds of substances, e.g. processed foods and carbonated beverages—that have wreaked so much havoc on our bodies in such a short span of time. Relying on our instincts to keep us healthy just doesn't work. We have to be that intelligent being, educate ourselves, use our higher brain and our logic, and figure it out for ourselves. No one can do this for us. Not a doctor, not a parent, not a spouse or well-intentioned friend. It's on each of us.

Your body is far smarter than you'll ever be. It's also the only one you've got and the only one you'll ever have. Sure, there are some artificial spare parts that work pretty well these days. As an orthopedist specializing in knees, my dad is one of the mechanics. But at the end of the day, the magnificent, living, breathing organism that is us is so incredible a design that it's pretty hard to improve upon it. You can't help but marvel at its beauty. I'm clearly not a poet. Plenty of those have put pen to paper and done a lot better job of describing the beauty of the human body than I could ever do, but the point I am trying to convey is that unless we get in the way of the body's most efficient functioning, it is pretty much of a masterpiece. It's when we don't care for and feed it properly that we run into trouble. While there is so much about the way our systems function that we don't know, what we do know is that if we don't feed our bodies lots of plant food, they're not going to operate as well and as for long as they should. It's that simple. The fuel I was putting into my body before the Reboot was not the fuel my engine ran best on. It still ran, but it was continually in the shop!

So what do I do now? Well, since my sixty-day Reboot I continue to Reboot for ten to fifteen days every three month. I do what I call a 5/5/5 Reboot, which consists of 15 days of consuming only fruit and vegetables.

The first and last 5 days are when I eat and drink them, and during the middle 5 I juice them. So over a twelve-month period, I have a whole two months when I'm living exclusively on plant food. My urticaria is in remission and I no longer take any medication whatsoever, I rarely if ever get sick anymore, and I generally feel energized and empowered. Are there times when I get off-track? Sure there are. I'm human. I might eat too much bread or over- indulge in ice-cream from time to time, but now that I know what it feels like to be clean and on top of my game, I now know how awful it feels when I'm not. My weight has stabilized around 220/230 lbs. That's 80/90 pounds lighter than when I set off on this adventure. I don't drink a lot of alcohol and I don't smoke anymore. I rarely eat animal protein and don't touch caffeine, except every now and then in chocolate, which still gets a good run for its money. That one is a work in progress....I'm much better than I used to be but there's always room for improvement. I don't touch soda anymore, I figure that one is just one of those things that I'll have to keep away from myself permanently.

As you can see, I'm not perfect. I don't know anyone who is. I'm also not about telling you what to eat. We are all unique. What my body can handle isn't necessarily what yours can. I don't think it's my place to tell you what not to eat. The last thing I would ever want to say to somebody was don't have that beer and hotdog at the ball game. My message is simply this: eat more plant food. Eat more fruit and vegetables. The more you eat, the better you'll feel. If you're up to the challenge and you really want to know what it's like to climb to the top of the mountain, try a Reboot. There's a lot in life I don't know, but this is one I know for sure: once you've got to the top of the mountain the view and the feeling is nothing short of amazing. The clarity of mind, the feeling of accomplishment, the pounds shed, the spring in your step and the love of life–these will change your outlook forever.

We live in a world of more than six billion people. In most places it's hard to go anywhere without rubbing elbows with another human, and yet as a people, we are measurably lonelier than we've ever been. What does that say about us? To me, it means that we lack a sense of community. In

Siong did a two-week Reboot to try and break her coffee habit, get rid of her migraines, and finally get some sleep.

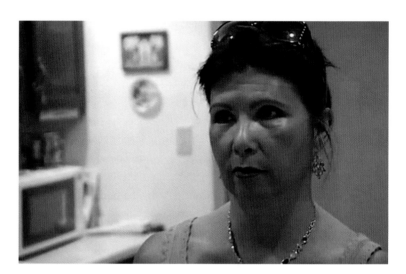

the past, meals were shared by a community of people who had made a team effort to grow, to hunt, to gather, to prepare our food; and who then sat together to enjoy the meal. But today, we have to work much harder to come together as a community.

Each person has a role to play. When you decide to press the reset button to Reboot, you'll need support. I felt this over and over when I traveled across the United States. I saw it with Phil Staples, who first reached out to me and then in turn supported so many others, both at the local organic market where he conducted community juice fasts and among his family and friends, especially his brother Bear.

I first met E Siong Norte, or Siong, as everyone calls her, on a visit to New York. She suffered terribly from migraine headaches, insomnia, moodiness, and lack of energy, and so we convinced her to give the Reboot a try. I don't think I've ever seen a person drink as much coffee in a day as she did, which was one of the habits she wanted to kick via the Reboot. She had the same relationship to coffee that I had with Coca-Cola. We Skyped regularly throughout her two-week Reboot, and talked via webcam, so I got to witness her gradual transformation. When she began the Reboot she looked drawn and exhausted, but by the end she was literally glowing. Her migraines disappeared. She began sleeping better. Her

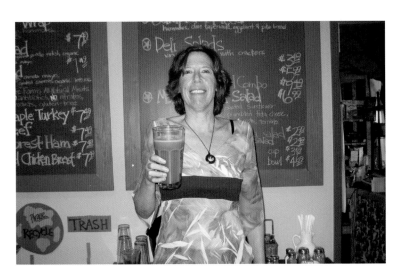

Tammy Hamlin, who was manager of the market in Iowa and inspired so many in her community.

energy level soared, and she started feeling very positive about life for the first time in awhile. I know Siong was amazed to discover how much power she could exercise over her health. She has permanently discovered the power of fruits and vegetables, and is one of the stars of the film.

For Tammy Hamlin, who managed the organic foods store in Spirit Lake called The Market, the place that became Phil Staples' second home, the idea of bringing people together via a community juice fast was, well, entirely natural. While Tammy has continued to support people in their efforts to get healthy, she has also continued her personal quest to get healthier. Tammy first tried Weight Watchers to lose weight, which was a step in the right direction, but she couldn't stay with it. Later, she decided to become a vegetarian, which helped her continue to lose weight and feel better. She eventually moved to Austin, Texas, where she found easy access to an abundance of good, healthy food, and where she met a lot of kindred souls who were as health-conscious as she was becoming. Tammy found that the healthier she ate, the more she wanted only healthy foods to eat. Fried foods and processed foods gave her a heavy, lethargic feeling, so she quit eating them altogether. The Reboot is, today, something she often recommends to friends and others who are in need of help on the health front.

I recently helped run a fifteen-day global Reboot. People from around the world, most of whom didn't even know each other, participated together. They connected online by blogging about their experiences, and reaching out to each other when they needed support or had questions. On Day Fifteen, this is what one of the participants had to say:

"WOW! I know everyone must be thinking/feeling some kind of amazement that it's here at last. It's been a journey, with ups and downs for sure. I feel like I took in a lot of information and moving forward, will approach food differently. I am VERY excited to be in a different place. I had been heading in a bad direction. For me it was the picking, the not thinking, the grabbing on the go, the not enjoying or chewing my food. The SUGAR and CAFFEINE and heavy, carby foods were tiring me out, giving me mood swings, and making me heavier than I wanted to be. So AMEN to the reboot. I feel rebooted!"

The question to ask yourself is: am I on track or off track? If you're on track, then keep on with whatever it is you're doing. If it ain't broke, why try and fix it? But if the answer is that you are off track, I know of no better way to Reboot your life and get back on track than by giving this a go. What it really comes down to is you. At the end of the day when the lights go out and you're alone in the house of mirrors, only you will be able to figure out how to fix things, and only you can make it happen. Change is a scary thing. It's stressful, it's the unknown. It's hard work. But in times of crisis, there is also opportunity. Seize the opportunity to make a change. I don't care how good or bad you've been to your body; it's never too late to Reboot. Your body has been there with you since Day One and it will do its best to self-repair and get back into great shape, if you give it a chance. Even if you have been rough on it for way too long don't fear, it will still do its best.

I know my simple, basic idea may still seem unreasonable, even crazy: nothing but juice. Nothing but fruit and vegetables. But I live by the following words and they have helped me through life when I've doubted myself, so I hope they help you. To paraphrase George Bernard Shaw:

The world is rarely changed by reasonable men (or women).

Juice On.

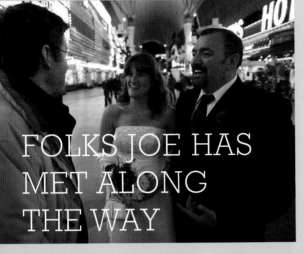

# FOLKS JOE HAS MET ALONG THE WAY

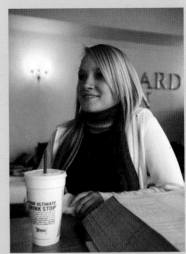

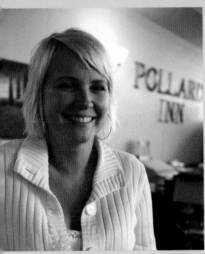

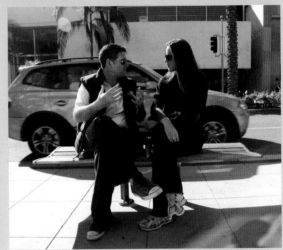

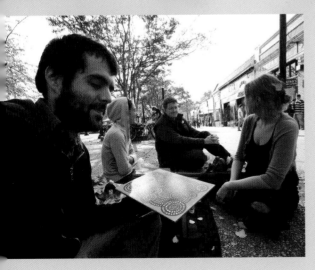

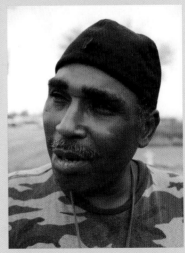

# CHAPTER ELEVEN

# NUTRITIONIST STACY KENNEDY IS YOUR PERSONAL REBOOT COACH: HOW TO REBOOT

I first met Stacy Kennedy when I visited Boston a few years ago, looking for advice on any possible link between my autoimmune condition and my diet.

Stacy holds multiple degrees and credentials relating to nutrition—MPH, RD, CSO and LDN. She is a Senior Clinical Nutritionist for Brigham and Women's Hospital/Dana-Farber Cancer Institute in Boston, and a board-certified specialist in oncology nutrition, as well as an integrative nutritionist with the Zakim Center for Integrative Therapies. She works in private practice too, including for my Reboot company, as Head Nutritionist. She is a big believer in the power of fruits and vegetables.

What follows is a chapter written by Stacy, in which she helps guide us through the practical aspects of the Reboot and educates us on some of the facts and science behind it.

When I first met Joe Cross and learned about his personal goals for better health and wellness, I knew right away that I had met someone who would be a great messenger for others. Joe was ready to make fundamental changes in his life, had done his homework, and was open to information and advice. Joe is used to being a leader, but he is one of those people who understands that he can't go everything alone. When he asked me to become a part of the Reboot team, counseling him on some of the practicalities of his own lifestyle changes and on how to present his message to a film audience and readers of his book, I knew he was offering me a unique opportunity. I jumped at the chance to share what I've learned in my own work at the Brigham and Women's Hospital/Dana-Farber Cancer Institute, where I am a senior clinical nutritionist. For this book, Joe wanted me to help readers move forward in their Reboots by providing some guidelines for them in the days leading up to the Reboot, during the period of the Reboot itself, and afterwards, when it is so important to continue to keep up the good work. That's where some of the hardest work begins.

As Joe has discussed throughout the book, juicing whole, fresh vegetables offers huge benefits. First of all, simply adding fresh fruit and vegetable juice to your daily diet is a great way to get healthier. Conducting an extended juice fast, or Reboot, can be a wonderful way to break bad eating habits, change food cravings, give your digestive system a rest from processed foods, and experience a stronger connection to yourself, your body, and your community. As Joe says, engaging in this kind of shift is a radical act.

Ideally, we would all eat raw and lightly cooked fruits and vegetables that are local, seasonal, fresh, and sometimes organic, PLUS juice. Whole produce and juiced produce are both important for different reasons. With whole fruits and vegetables we get lots of vitamins, minerals, phytonutrients, and fiber. With juicing, we also get an abundance of vitamins, minerals, and phytonutrients, but because the food has been liquefied, it is easier for our systems to absorb the nutrients more efficiently and for us to consume more of them at once.

What follows is a kind of roadmap to help you prepare a program of consuming fruit and vegetables, which may or may not include a short-term juice fast to "reboot" your system and begin your journey to optimal health. In this section, you will also find some helpful science, some recipes, and other information to support your post-Reboot, healthy-eating lifestyle. We recommend three different Reboot programs: 5 or 15 days of eating fruits and vegetables PLUS drinking fresh juice once or twice a day, as described in the Reboot Express and the Reboot Entry programs, respectively. The third program is the Reboot Standard, or 5-5-5 you learned about earlier in the book—5 days of eating fruits and vegetables plus juicing once or twice a day, 5 days of just juicing, then 5 days of eating and juicing just like the first 5 days.

Once you have made the choice to go on your five or fifteen-day Reboot, you should you should mentally and practically prepare yourself for what you may encounter along the way. Anticipate that there will be periods when you will be very tired, when you will feel isolated or lonely, when you might question why you are putting yourself through all this. Make it easier on yourself by setting aside some downtime when you can pamper yourself if possible, even just staying in bed for a day if you feel like it and can get help with your other responsibilities. However, keep in mind that sticking to a juice fast can be much tougher during the holidays or other celebratory times. As surprisingly delicious as you will find the freshly made fruit and vegetable juices to be, who wants to be the only one in the room having to refuse every item of food offered that is not juice? It is also best to do as much of your produce shopping as you can prior to the start of the Reboot so you don't find yourself on that first day, when you may be very low on energy, having to run out to the market in order to make your first "meal."

During the juicing days of your Reboot, if you follow the 5-5-5 program, you're going to be drinking approximately 64 ounces of fresh fruit and vegetable juice per day, supplemented by filtered water or other non-caffeinated beverages such as herbal teas or coconut water for variety. But you won't be consuming any "solid" foods.

# MICRO, MACRO, AND PHYTONUTRIENTS

The average American eats 2.5 servings of fruits and vegetables combined each day.

Only 23% of Americans get the recommended 5 or more servings a day.

Painful, chronic conditions such as constipation, irritable bowel syndrome, migraines, chronic fatigue syndrome and fibromyalgia could be alleviated through adopting a plant-based, micronutrient-rich diet.

Complex foods can be grouped into two major categories—macronutrients and micronutrients. Both groups work together to keep our bodies running smoothly; without the right balance of micronutrients, all the protein in the world won't allow us to build muscle effectively.

Macronutrients are elements like carbohydrates, proteins, and fats that we need, but should not consume in excess.

Micronutrients include all vitamins, minerals, and phytonutrients. Phytonutrients, which comprise the plant's immune system, have properties that can defend our bodies against the toxic environments we live in.

Phytonutrients and micronutrients are found in all plant-based foods, including fruits, vegetables, whole grains, spices, herbs, and teas.

To date, there are thousands of micronutrient phytonutrients that have been identified in plants, such as carotenes, antioxidants, and flavonoids. Often we hear that the vitamin C in an orange is responsible for its immune-boosting properties, but there are actually over 170 known phytonutrients in just one orange! To get over a cold more quickly eat plenty of citrus fruits, especially oranges.

Fruits and vegetables highest in phenoilcs, a group of micronutrients with potent health benefits, include cranberry, apple, red grapes, strawberry, pineapple, banana, peach, lemon, orange, pear, grapefruit, broccoli, spinach, onion, and red pepper.

Oxidative damage is linked to the formation of tumors. Eating fruits and vegetables high in antioxidants will prevent too much oxidative stress from taking a toll on the body.

## PREPARING FOR THE REBOOT

I am going to break out the preparation steps for your Reboot into into ten parts:

STEP 1: Purchase a good quality juicer. There are many on the market at a variety of price points. Some are easier to clean than others, you'll notice. We recommend juicers that remove fiber. You can educate yourself on the right juicer for you by reading up on various juicers online, or calling the company directly to ask questions.

STEP 2: Identify the most affordable, convenient source of local, seasonal produce before you officially start your juice fast. Be sure to wash all your produce well before juicing, including any stems or leaves, using cold, running water and a brush.

STEP 3: Well before the start of Reboot, begin incorporating some fresh juice into your diet, at least one serving a day.

STEP 4: If you have any food allergies or sensitivities, be sure you keep a list of them handy when choosing produce.

STEP 5: Two weeks prior to the start of your Reboot, start to eliminate all processed junk foods, white flour, sugar, fried food, fast food, processed meats (e.g. ham, salami, bologna, bacon, sausage, hot dogs, etc.), and alcohol from your diet. Begin to reduce your caffeine intake, so that by the end of the first week you are off it altogether.

STEP 6: Steadily add more and more salads, soups, fruit and vegetable smoothies, whole grains, nuts, seeds, nut butters, beans, and legumes to your diet on a daily basis during the two weeks prior to the start of your Reboot.

STEP 7: In terms of animal protein, consume only wild-caught fish or organic eggs during this period. If you are eating poultry, be sure it is organic and gradually reduce your consumption of it so that by Day Eleven of the two-week countdown you're down to zero poultry.

STEP 8: Your intake of red meat should end completely by Day Four of the countdown leading up to your Reboot. By the time you start the Reboot, all of your protein should be coming exclusively from plant sources.

STEP 9: Consume only low or non-fat organic dairy with little to no added sugars, or unflavored soy, rice or almond milk for the first few days of the countdown.

STEP 10: By day five of the period preceding the Reboot, all dairy should be gone from your diet.

## DURING THE REBOOT

### LIQUIDS

Even though you will be drinking about 64 oz of fresh juice daily during the juicing phase of your 5-5-5 Reboot, you will need to supplement to meet your hydration needs. Most beverages that don't contain caffeine, sugar, or alcohol are hydrating: herbal teas, ginger root tea with lemon, coconut water, or just plain filtered water are some good examples.

If you are constipated, excessively tired, in a hot climate, at a higher altitude, engaging in strenuous activity, visiting a sauna, doing hot yoga, heavier or taller than average, or used to drinking 3-4 liters or quarts of water a day, you may have greater fluid requirements and should make an extra effort to make sure you are staying hydrated.

### FRUIT v. VEGETABLE JUICE

Strive to limit your intake of fruit-only juice primarily to the morning, though of course, you can always add a vegetable or two to the morning juice as desired. For the rest of the day, your juice should be comprised mostly of vegetables—about 80% veggies and 20% fruits. While adding a little fruit to the vegetable juice is a great way to improve its taste, if you rely too heavily on fruits you'll miss out on the wealth of micronutrients locked away in vegetables. Also, drinking a substantial amount of fruit juice can lead to rapid sugar absorption, a resulting energy crash, and a spike in insulin, which is an inflammation-promoting hormone we need to metabolize sugar.

## Frequently Asked Questions:

### 1. WHAT IF A REBOOT ISN'T RIGHT FOR ME RIGHT NOW?

If you are pregnant or nursing; undergoing dialysis, chemotherapy, or radiation; are underweight or in active therapy for an eating disorder; have uncontrolled diabetes, epilepsy, low blood pressure, liver disease, anemia, impaired immune function, ulcerative colitis, Crohn's disease, or other autoimmune disorders, a Reboot is not recommended. However, even under these conditions (with the exception of pregnant or lactating women), you may be able to embark on a modified Reboot under a physician's supervision. If you have a chronic health condition; have been sick with a cold, flu, or other infection; take medications daily, or are very young or elderly, please take extra care to speak with your physician before starting a Reboot. But even if your physician does not advise a Reboot for you right now, don't despair. You can still begin to follow a diet that includes more fruits and vegetables. If you are planning to add juice to your existing diet, drinking 8-16 ounces per day is recommended.

### 2. WHAT ABOUT WEIGHT LOSS?

Weight loss is a typical side effect of a Reboot, which for some is great news. You will most likely lose weight due to the fact that you are ingesting fewer calories than usual and using stores of protein and fats to keep your brain and normal bodily functions working. It is natural for a little weight to come back on after the Reboot period, even if afterwards you continue to maintain a healthy, micronutrient-rich diet. Try not to be discouraged, though: by following a well designed, calorie controlled, micronutrient-rich eating plan, your healthy weight loss can continue after the Reboot. Visit our website www.jointhereboot.com to learn how to construct your personalized, micronutrient-based, weight management plan.

### 3. WHAT ARE THE BENEFITS OF USING ORGANIC v. CONVENTIONAL PRODUCE?

Studies have shown that certain organic foods have higher levels of nutrients than conventionally grown foods, although whether they are better for us or will make a difference in preventing diseases remains to be determined. At the same time, there is ample evidence about the potential negative health effects of the pesticides consumed by the general U.S. population along with our food. It is important to note, however, that most of the research showing the benefits of eating fruits and vegetables is either based on conventional produce, or does not distinguish between who ate organic and who did not. The bottom line is that it's best to eat more produce—organic or not—and wash it well, because the benefits of eating fresh fruits and vegetables outweigh the risks associated with pesticide residue.

Below are some guidelines developed by the Environmental Working Group and the USDA to help to help you choose which foods to buy organic when possible.

| Produce with highest levels of pesticide residue: choose organic for these | Produce with lowest levels of pesticide residue: less need to choose organic |
|---|---|
| Peach | Onion |
| Apples | Avocado |
| Bell Peppers (green & red) | Sweet Corn |
| Celery | Pineapple |
| Nectarine | Mango |
| Strawberries | Asparagus |
| Cherries | Sweet Peas |
| Kale | Kiwi |
| Lettuce | Cabbage |
| Grapes (imported) | Eggplant |
| Carrot | Papaya |
| Pear | Watermelon |
| Potato | Broccoli |

Organic foods are also more expensive than conventional foods, as much as 50 to 100% more. Finding affordable organic or no/low-spray produce can be possible with a little research and planning.

## 4.  WHAT TIME OF YEAR IS BEST FOR A REBOOT?

Some people find it easier to be on a Reboot when the weather is warmer. Winter may not be the ideal, as going on a juice fast can lower the body's temperature. The ideal place to go on a Reboot is in an environment of fresh air, clean water, lots of sun, and low stress levels. Of course, this is not where most of us live, so we need to just do the best we can. See if you can adapt your home environment to include some items from this "optimal" list by utilizing meditation, yoga, prayer, or gardening to help promote stress reduction. If you have access to the ocean or mountains, hiking trails, state parks, or other outdoor venues, take advantage of them during your Reboot. Even a walk around your neighborhood or local parks will be beneficial.

## 5.  WHAT'S THE DIFFERENCE BETWEEN JUICING AND DRINKING PRE-PACKAGED, COMMERCIAL JUICES?

Most commercial juices lack the nutritional value of freshly juiced fruits and vegetables. Many juices on the market have more sugar per ounce than soda! Those that have 100% juice are obviously better than those with only 10%. However, all varieties of commercial juice entail processing and travel, thereby decreasing the amounts of nutrients and enzymes they contain.

# JUICING TIPS

* Wash fruits or vegetables thoroughly.
* Line juicer's pulp basket with a plastic bag for easy clean-up.
* Cut or tear produce into pieces that will fit in juicer.
* Each juice should be at least 16 oz.
* Lemon, Lime, or Ginger root can be added to any juice.

# SUGGESTED JUICING MENU AND SCHEDULE

### First thing in the morning
Hot water with Lemon, plus a separate glass of water, at least 16 oz.

### Morning Juice: Apple-Pear
1 Apple
2 Pears
1 piece Ginger (thumb-sized)

### Mid-Morning Juice: Carrot-Kale Combo
1 Green Apple
3 handfuls Spinach
6-8 Kale leaves
4 large Carrots
1 piece Ginger (thumb-sized)

### Mid-Aftenoon Juice: Kale-Cucumber-Celery

1 Green Apple

3 handfuls Spinach

6-8 Kale leaves

½ Cucumber

4 Celery stalks

½ Lemon

### Evening Juice: Carrot-Apple-Beet

1 Apple

2 Beets

3 large Carrots

1 piece Ginger (thumb-sized)

3 handfuls Spinach

6-8 Kale leaves

### Night

Herbal Tea

Write in your journal about the day's experiences.

## Fruits and Vegetables Commonly Used in Juicing.

KALE: An especially nutrient-dense vegetable that is rich in calcium, lutein, iron, and vitamins A, C, and K. Kale has seven times the beta-carotene of broccoli and ten times more lutein, another potent carotene. Carotenes act as antioxidants and may help protect against cancer. Kale is also a cruciferous vegetable (see box below).

CELERY: High in organic sodium, magnesium, and iron. Magnesium is important for the breakdown of carbohydrates, proteins, and fats into energy. It also aids muscle relaxation and prevention of muscle cramps, nerve conduction, and the prevention of tooth decay.

CUCUMBER: Contains potassium and phytosterols, which help lower blood cholesterol levels.

PARSLEY: Good source of folate, which may help lower the risk of heart disease and certain types of cancers. Also promotes fresh breath.

SPINACH: High in iron, vitamin C, and beta-carotene, which are antioxidants and may help to protect cells from the damaging effects of free radicals.

CARROT: The richest plant source of vitamin A, good source of potassium

BEET: Packed with potent antioxidants, liver-protective properties.

CILANTRO: Rich source of carotenoids.

CABBAGE: A cruciferous vegetable promoting natural detoxification. High in sulfur and iodine.

APPLE: Naturally high in antioxidants that help protect "good" HDL cholesterol levels in the blood.

**LEMON:** Contains natural anti-nausea and overall digestive aid properties

**PINEAPPLE:** High in the enzyme bromelain, this acts as an anti-inflammatory.

**KIWI:** Twice the vitamin C of an orange. Good source of vitamin E (a potent antioxidant) and potassium.

**GINGER ROOT:** Reduces nausea and heartburn, pain and inflammation. Aids digestion.

**SWISS CHARD:** Tastes sweeter in juices than spinach. Rich in vitamin C, potassium, and magnesium. Foods rich in potassium have been shown to lower blood pressure and the risk of heart disease.

DO NOT JUICE:
Sprouts
Figs
Bananas
Avocado
Bok Choy

## CRUCIFEROUS VEGETABLES: NATURAL DETOXIFIERS

Broccoli, cauliflower, cabbage, brussel sprouts, kale, radish, and wasabi are cruciferous vegetables, which increase the enzymes that give our liver more detox capability. It is important to choose one serving each day from this family. Some people may not want to juice these vegetables because they are gas-producing. However, small amounts of red cabbage or broccoli can often be juiced without problem.

WHAT
COUNTS AS A
SERVING?

1 cup
leafy greens,
berries or
melon chunks

½ cup
cut or cooked
fruits and
vegetables
(broccoli,
carrots,
pineapple...)

1 medium
piece of fruit
or vegetable
(apple, plum,
peach, orange)

6 ounces
natural, fresh
100% fruit/
vegetable
juice

¼ cup
dried fruit
(sulfur free)

BEYOND THE REBOOT
(this guide can also help you boost the amount
of micronutrients in your everyday diet).

Now that you've completed your Reboot, you can gently and gradually transition to digesting more complex foods. Avoid fast food, packaged foods, and high-fat foods: after five to fifteen days of fresh fruit and vegetable juice, your body will not be happy if you eat them and the result will likely be stomach pain, bloating, indigestion, and fatigue.

Here are some overall suggestions for planning your meals for the first, post-Reboot week.

Choose as many local, seasonal, organic foods as possible.

Begin by adding whole fruits and vegetables. Avoid raw, gas-producing vegetables, like brussel sprouts, broccoli, cauliflower, and cabbage for the first few days.

Eat smaller amounts more often. This will be essential to retraining your digestive system to process complex combinations of foods.

Salads, smoothies, and soups made from fresh, seasonal, local and/or organic produce are excellent ways to both prepare for and ramp down from the Reboot, as well as to boost the variety of micronutrient-rich foods in your diet. Invest in a good quality blender and food processor (many are sold as combos or with attachments for both).

SALADS should include a variety of colors, textures, and flavors to improve taste and increase the amount of wholesome micronutrients. Add ingredients such as lentils, organic soybeans, black beans, quinoa and wheat berries, as well as tofu, edamame, and nuts.

SMOOTHIES are a healthy breakfast or snack. Begin your smoothie by adding fresh vegetable/fruit juice to some type of milky product, such as low-fat organic milk or yogurt, almond or hemp milk, organic soy milk, or coconut water. Then add whole fruits, fresh or frozen. Frozen, organic fruit will make your smoothie cold and add more nutrients than ice. Bananas are excellent for thickening up a smoothie.

SOUPS are a great way to warm up with nutrient-packed, light food (and cold soups such as avocado or gazpacho can be a pleasurable addition to your diet in warm weather). Homemade soups can also help remedy digestive challenges brought on by eating a large amount of raw vegetables. Start with a vegetable broth, then add lots and lots of veggies (use frozen vegetables for items out of season in your area). Even though vegetables in soups are cooked for a long time, the soup retains much of the fresh, raw vegetables' original nutrient content. While the water-soluble vitamins decrease within the actual vegetable, most "fall off" into the liquid of the soup, which gives you these vital nutrients when you consume it. And don't forget about adding lentils or black/kidney beans.

### EAT BY THE RAINBOW.

Choosing one fruit or vegetable from each color family is another good way to get your five servings a day.

RED: tomato, watermelon, red pepper, beets
ORANGE/YELLOW: orange, sweet potato, mango, winter squash
DARK GREEN: spinach, kale, swiss chard, mustard greens,
collard greens
BLUE/PURPLE: blueberries, eggplant, concord grapes,
purple cabbage
SOY FOODS: edamame, tofu, soy milk

## The 4 Ps: Plants, Proteins, Planning, and Preparation

PLANTS: Your goal for a healthy daily diet should be to eat at least 5 daily servings of fruits and vegetables. It is often recommended that this consist of 3 or more servings of vegetables and 2 servings of fruits a day, but both Dr. Fuhrman and I think we need more vegetables than fruits to maximize the benefit of a micronutrient-rich diet. 5 or more servings a day may sound like a lot of food, but it's really not. For example:

Over the 2 cups (AUS 1.5 cups) of greens in a salad, toss on ¼ cup of carrots, ¼ cup of cucumber, ¼ cup of broccoli, ¼ cup of peppers, (AUS, slightly more than ⅛ cup), and you've got 4 servings!

In a smoothie, blend ½ banana, 1 cup blueberries, 1 cup strawberries, and already you're more than halfway to your goal of at least 5 a day.

PROTEINS: The majority of proteins in your diet should be plant-based.

Nuts, seeds, nut butters (such as almond, sunflower seed, soynut, peanut, cashew)

Beans and legumes (such as hummus, black beans, white beans, kidney beans, lentils) and soy foods (edamame, soy milk, tofu, tempeh).

For animal proteins, choose wild-caught fish, organic eggs, and organic poultry. If you eat red meat choose lean, grass-fed, organic meats, including bison, buffalo, and ostrich in addition to beef. Red meat should be consumed sparingly, 6-8 ounces a week.

Choose organic, low-fat dairy products.

PLANNING: Eating on a set schedule will help your system resume a healthy, balanced diet, and is the key to managing hunger and satiety. A small, frequent meal pattern is essential for reaping the benefits of a micronutrient-rich healthy lifestyle. Maintaining your schedule and diet takes some planning ahead;

Look up restaurant menus online to review choices before going out to eat.

Bring portable, micronutrient-rich snacks with you on the go.

Eat breakfast at home before going out for the day.

Bring your lunch and 1-2 snacks to work/school.

Don't go grocery shopping when you're hungry.

Shop the perimeter of the grocery store to stock up on micronutrients.

## PREPARING HEALTHY MEALS

What is the best way to cook micronutrient-rich foods? Let's review a few cooking techniques to help you make this a permanent lifestyle change.

BAKING: Place food in the oven in either a covered or uncovered glass baking dish, a baking sheet, or other oven-safe cookware.

BROILING: Use your oven to cook at a higher temperature. This is a great alternative to frying for giving food a crisp outside that approximates grilling. Avoid charring or overcooking animal proteins, which creates carcinogens.

GRILLING: An outdoor version of broiling. Charred vegetables do not carry carcinogens (they have different protein structures), so there is no harm in charring peppers on the grill for a sweet flavor.

ROASTING: Similar to baking, but at higher temperatures. A baking sheet or roasting pan is best. Roasting on parchment paper is a great way to cook vegetables.

STEAMING: Use a steamer or place a steaming basket over simmering liquid on the stove. Lightly steam vegetables so they maintain their color and crispness.

STIR-FRYING: Use a small amount of oil in a non-teflon, non-stick pan or wok on the stovetop. Rapidly stir small pieces of food with a wooden spoon or BPA-free plastic spatula to lightly cook and maintain natural color and texture. Also great for cooking organic/cage-free chicken.

# RECIPES

From Jointhereboot.com

# SALADS

### Reboot Green Salad

Use any greens (romaine hearts, baby romaine, baby spinach, baby arugula), along with any veggie (cucumber, carrot, celery, pepper, tomato, fennel, radish, red onion), and fresh herbs (cilantro, basil). Avocado, edamame, walnuts, wheat berries & dried cranberries may also be added for more substance.

### Ginger Honey Soy Dressing

Minced Fresh Ginger (US 2 Tbsp, AUS ¾ Tbsp or 2dsp plus 2 tsp)
Minced Fresh Garlic (US 2 Tbsp, AUS ¾ Tbsp or 2dsp plus 2 tsp)
Raw Honey (US 2 Tbsp, AUS ¾ Tbsp or 2dsp plus 2 tsp)
Nama Shoyu or Tamari (US 4Tbsp, AUS 3 Tbsp or 4dsp plus 4 tsp)
Olive Oil (US 4Tbsp, AUS 3 Tbsp or 4dsp plus 4 tsp)

Puree the first four ingredients in a blender. With the blender running, slowly add the oil until the dressing is emulsified. Keeps up to a week in the refrigerator.

# SMOOTHIES

### Blackberry Kiwi Blend

¼ large Pineapple, core removed and roughly cubed
Blackberries (US 1 cup, AUS ¾ cup and 2 Tbsp plus 1 dsp)
1 Kiwi Fruit
1 Banana
½ Comice Pear
Coconut Water (US 1 cup, AUS 125 ml)
30 Mint leaves
Flax Seed Oil (US 1 Tbsp, AUS ¾ Tbsp or 1 dsp plus 1 tsp)

Add all ingredients to blender and liquefy.

# SOUPS

## Vegetable Soup

Olive Oil (US 3 Tbsp, AUS 2 ¼ Tbsp or 3 dsp plus 3 tsp)

1 large Onion, chopped

3 cloves Garlic, minced

3 medium Carrots, chopped

3 Celery Stalks, chopped

3 Tomatoes, chopped with juice reserved

1 medium Zucchini, cut into half moons

Green Beans, trimmed to 1-inch or 2.5 cm pieces
    (US 1 cup, AUS ¾ cup)

3-4 handfuls Kale or other leafy green, such as Chard or Bok Choy, chopped into small pieces

Water (US 6 cups, AUS 1,500 ml)

fresh Thyme, chopped (US ¾ Tbsp, AUS 2 and ¼ Tbsp)

fresh Oregano (US 1 Tbsp, AUS ¾ Tbsp plus 1 dsp)

freshly ground Black Pepper (US 1 tsp, AUS 1 tsp)

In a large stock pot, heat the olive oil over medium high heat. Add the onion, garlic, carrots, and celery and sauté for 5 minutes. Add the tomatoes, zucchini, green beans, water, salt, pepper, thyme, and oregano; stir and bring to a boil. Redue the heat to a simmer and cook for 10 minutes. Add the chopped kale or other leafy greens and cook for an additional 5 minutes. Season to taste with the salt and pepper.

## Sweet Potato and Bok Choy Soup

Olive Oil (US 3 Tbsp, AUS 2 ¼ Tbsp or 3 dsp and 3 tsp)

1 medium Onion, diced

2 Leeks, white part only, roughly chopped

2 cloves Garlic, minced

a pinch of Red Pepper Flakes

2 medium Carrots, sliced into rounds

2 Celery Stalks, diced

1 large Sweet Potato, peeled and roughly chopped

2 sprigs Thyme

2 sprigs Parsley

Salt (US 1 tsp, AUS 1 tsp)

Water (US 4 cups, AUS 1 liter)

1 large Bok Choy or 3 Baby Bok Choy, cleaned and torn into pieces

freshly ground Black Pepper (US ½ tsp, AUS ½ tsp)

Heat the oil in a large pot over medium heat. Add the onion, leeks, garlic, and red pepper flakes and sauté until the vegetables soften, about 3 minutes.

Add the carrots, celery, sweet potato, thyme, parsley, and salt and sauté 3 minutes. Add the water and increase the heat to high. Bring the mixture to a boil, then return to a simmer and cook until the vegetables soften, about 30 minutes. Stir in the bok choy and cook for another 5 minutes. Stir in the pepper and any additional salt if necessary.

Remove the thyme and parsley sprigs and serve.

# VEGETABLES

### Roasted Veggies—Mushroom, Eggplant, Sweet Potato, Kale

6 Portabella Mushroom Caps or 1 package Baby Bella Mushrooms

1 Eggplant

1 medium Sweet Potato

1 Onion

8-10 leaves Kale

3 cloves Garlic

1 pinch Paprika

freshly ground Black Pepper (US ⅛ tsp, AUS ⅛ tsp)

Mustard Seed (US ⅛ tsp, AUS ⅛ tsp)

ground Cumin (US ¼ tsp, AUS ¼ tsp)

Preheat oven to 450 degrees Fahrenheit/230 degrees Celsius.

Wash all ingredients well (except onion). Cut into medium-sized wedges. Place on parchment paper. Spray with Olive Oil, add seasonings.

Roast in oven for approximately 20-30 minutes. Add kale for the last 5 minutes.

Place into bowl, squeeze garlic onto other veggies.

## Baked Zucchini with Tomatoes and Herbs

3 small Zucchini

4 Schallions, sliced, white and green parts separated

1 small Onion, chopped

2 Plum Tomatoes, coarsely chopped

Celery Leaves (from inner stalks), chopped (US 2 Tbsp, AUS 2 ½ Tbsp or 2 dsp and 2 tsp)

Basil Leaves, chopped, plus extra for garnish (US 4 Tbsp, AUS 3 Tbsp)

Olive Oil (US ¼ cup, AUS 3 Tbsp or 63 ml)

Sea Salt (US 1 tsp. AUS 1 tsp)

freshly ground Black Pepper (US ½ tsp, AUS ½ tsp)

Preheat oven to 425 degrees Fahrenheit/220 degrees Celsius. Slice the zucchini in half crosswise. Cut each half again lengthwise, then slice each of the halves into 4 equal, ½-inch or 1 cm pieces. They should look like sticks.

In a bowl, mix together the zucchini sticks with the white parts of the scallions, onion, tomatoes, celery leaves, and basil. Mix in the olive oil, salt, and pepper and toss to combine.

Pour into a 3-quart baking dish and bake for 20 minutes. Garnish with the sliced green tops of the scallions and the extra chopped basil.

## Cauliflower Mash

2 heads cauliflower

Olive oil

Sea salt and pepper

Other spices to taste

Preheat oven to 425 Fahrenheit/220 degrees Celsius. Trim cauliflower down to florets. Roast half of the cauliflower in the oven for 20-25 minutes, turning florets once during roasting. Steam remaining cauliflower for 6 minutes. Mash or puree steamed cauliflower. Chop roasted cauliflower into small chunks, mix in with the mashed. Season to taste.

# AFTERWORD BY
# DEAN ORNISH, M.D.

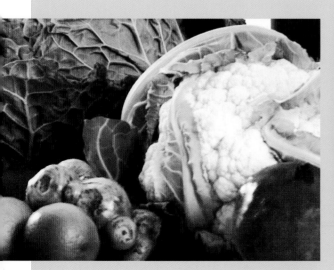
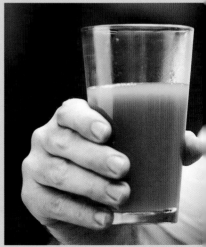

By now, you may have finished reading *Fat, Sick, & Nearly Dead*. I hope you found it to be as inspiring as I did.

Joe Cross's story powerfully illustrates an important point: our bodies often have a remarkable capacity to begin healing, and more quickly than had once been thought possible, if we simply stop doing what's causing the problem. In many cases, the lifestyle choices we make are powerful determinants of our health and well-being.

When I lecture, I frequently show a slide of doctors busily mopping up the floor around a sink that's overflowing, but no one is turning off the faucet. When we address the causes of our suffering, our bodies often can begin to heal.

Many people tend to think of breakthroughs in medicine as a new drug, laser, or high-tech surgical procedure. They often have a hard time believing that the simple choices that we make in our lifestyle—what we eat, how we respond to stress, whether or not we smoke cigarettes, how much exercise we get, and the quality of our loving relationships and social support—can be as powerful as drugs and surgery, but they often are. Sometimes, even better.

For more than 34 years, I have directed a series of studies showing what a powerful difference changes in diet and lifestyle can make. My colleagues and I at the non-profit Preventive Medicine Research Institute showed that what was once thought to be impossible was often achievable. We used high-tech, state-of-the-art measures to prove the power of simple, low-tech, and low-cost interventions.

We showed, for the first time, that many diseases, including coronary heart disease and early-stage prostate cancer, are often reversible and thus largely preventable, as well as type 2 diabetes, high blood pressure, high cholesterol levels, obesity, depression, and even some forms of cancer. The need for drugs and surgery is often greatly reduced when people make comprehensive lifestyle changes.

Our latest research showed that changing your lifestyle changes your genes in only three months—turning on hundreds of genes that prevent disease and turning off genes and turning off oncogenes that promote breast cancer, prostate cancer, and colon cancer as well as genes that cause heart disease, oxidative stress, and inflammation. We also found that these lifestyle changes increase telomerase, the enzyme that lengthens telomeres, the ends of our chromosomes that control how long we live. Even drugs have not been shown to do this.

So often, I hear people say, "Oh, it's all in my genes, there's not much I can do about it," which I call "genetic nihilism." It's empowering to know that your genes are a predisposition, but your genes are not your fate. Health care costs—really, sick care costs—are reaching a tipping point in which they often exceed net revenues for many corporations. Heart disease, diabetes, prostate/breast cancer, and obesity account for 75% of health care costs, and yet these are largely preventable and even reversible by changing diet and lifestyle.

I've found that sustainable changes in lifestyle are based on pleasure, abundance, and freedom. What you *include* in your diet is as important as what you *exclude*. And there's no point in giving up something that you enjoy unless you get something back that's even better—and quickly.

Life is to be fully enjoyed.

Because the mechanisms that affect our health are so much more dynamic than had once been realized, most people find that when they make the lifestyle changes described in this book, they feel so much better, so quickly. This reframes the reason for change from fear of dying (which is not sustainable) to joy of living (which is). It's not just about preventing illness or living *longer*; it's about living *better*.

When you eat and live healthier, your brain gets more blood so you think more clearly, have more energy, need less sleep. You can even grow so many new brain cells that your brain can get measurably bigger in just a few months! Your skin gets more blood so you wrinkle less and look younger. Your sexual organs get more blood flow in the same way that drugs like Viagra work, so you enhance sexual potency.

In our studies, we found that the more people changed, the better they felt and the more they improved in ways we could measure. And the better they felt, the more motivated they were to continue. The primary determinant of improvement was not how old they were or how sick they were; it was how much they changed their lifestyle.

If you're dealing with a life-threatening illness like Joe, then it makes sense to eat and live on the healthiest end of the spectrum—the "pound of cure." Moderate changes may not be enough to reverse a life-threatening illness like heart disease. But many people who are not dealing with a life-threatening condition aren't ready to make a complete Reboot, and it's important to start where you are and do what you can. Be compassionate with yourself.

You have a spectrum of choices; it's not all or nothing. If you indulge yourself one day, eat healthier the next. If you forget to exercise one day, do a little more the next. If you don't have time to meditate for a half hour, meditate for one minute. You get the idea.

In addition to the health benefits, choosing *not* to do something that we otherwise could do helps define who we are, reminds us that we have free will, freedom of choice. Only when we can say "no" are we free to say "yes."

That's what the most enlightened spiritual teachers have taught through the millennia: how to live a joyful life, right here and now. There are ways of living in the world that make it a lot more fun and happy.

In this context, what we choose to eat—and not eat—can nourish our soul as well as our body. Each meal reminds us that our lives can be much more than they are. Any time we can make what we do more special and meaningful, it becomes more fun.

All religions have dietary restrictions, but they differ from one another. Whatever the intrinsic benefit in eating or avoiding certain foods, just the act of choosing not to eat or not to do something that we otherwise might be able to helps to make our lives more sacred, more special, more disciplined, more meaningful.

When we consciously choose to limit what we're doing, it liberates us. Discipline can be liberating if it's freely chosen rather than imposed, because it enables us to do things and to express ourselves in ways that we otherwise might not be able to do. For example, musicians practicing scales may feel it's a little tedious at times, but it enables them to express themselves more freely by playing beautiful music.

In this context, choosing to eat and live differently can be a joyful spiritual practice rather than one leaving you feeling deprived or depressed. We can enjoy life more fully by making these conscious choices. Love is more sustainable than fear.

Awareness is the first step in healing. Science is a powerful way of raising awareness, and stories like Joe's can be healing as well.

**Dean Ornish, M.D.**
**Founder and President, Preventive Medicine Research Institute**
**Clinical Professor of Medicine, University of California, San Francisco**
**www.pmri.org**

# ABOUT THE AUTHOR

Joe Cross is an Australian entrepreneur and businessman. He attended high school at St Ignatius College, Riverview, in Australia, where he received a Jesuit education. The most important lesson he took away from school was the Jesuit admonition that one must be "Men for Others."

Without first going to college, Joe went to work as a clerk on the floor of the Sydney Futures Exchange, rising to become a successful Local Member, which is another way of saying that you're making trades using your own money. In 1994 at the age of 28, Joe founded his first company. Since that time, he has worked as a serial entrepreneur, enjoying the benefits of building businesses and getting to work with fabulous people. It's Joe's belief that if you're not getting the appreciation you deserve, or continuing to learn in your job, then it's time to leave or make a change!

Since 2007 after successfully selling the company he founded thirteen years before, he shifted his focus to the Health and Wellness space, producing and directing the film FAT, SICK & NEARLY DEAD, and launching the company Reboot Holdings.

He is Chairman and majority stakeholder in Reboot Holdings. Joe remains determined to eat more fruits and vegetables than he used to, and hopes that others will follow.

This is his first book.

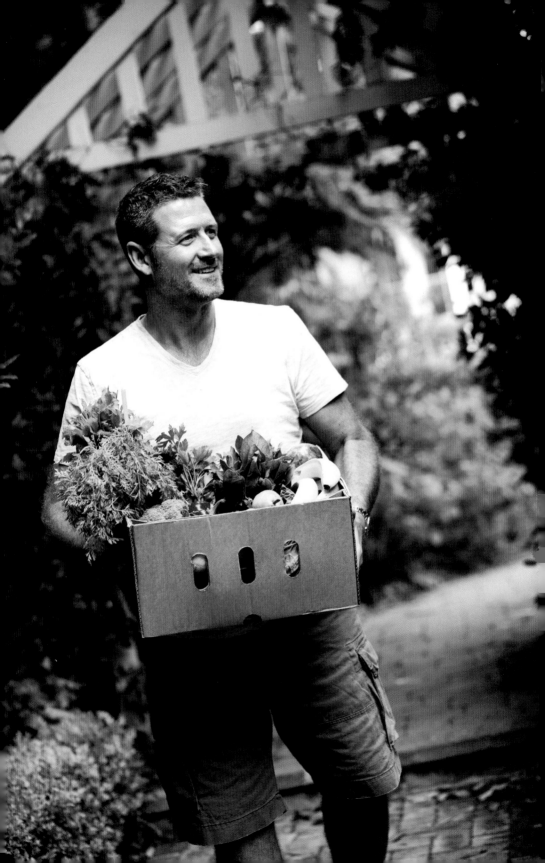

## ADDITIONAL REFERENCES:

From beginning doc:

1. Reeves MJ, Rafferty AP. Healthy Lifestyle Characteristics Among Adults in the United States, 2000. Arch Intern Med. 2005;165:854-857s

2. Joshipura, KJ, Hu, RB, Manson, JE, et al. The effect of fruit and vegetable intake on risk for coronary heart disease. Ann Intern Med 2001;134:1106.

3. Bazzano, LA, He, J, Ogden, LG, et al. Legume consumption and risk of coronary heart disease in US men and women: NHANES I Epidemiologic Gollfow-up Study. Arch Intern Med 2001;161:2573.

4. He, FJ, Nowson, CA, MacGregor, GA. Fruit and vegetable consumption and stroke: meta-analysis of cohort studies. Lancet 2006;367:320.

5. Joshipura, KJ, Hu, RB, Manson, JE, et al. Fruit and vegetable intake in relation to risk of ischemic stroke. JAMA 1999;282:1233.

6. Gillman, MW, Cupples, LA, Gagnon, D, et al. Protective effect of fruits and vegetables on development of stroke in men. JAMA 16995;273:1113.

7. Ascherio, A, Rimm, EB, Hernan, MA, eg al. Intake of potassium, magnesium, calcium, and fiber and risk of stroke among US men. Circulation 1998;98:1198.

8. Ford ES, Bergmann MM, Kroger J, Schienkiewitz A, Weikert C, Boeing H. Healthy Living Is the Best Revenge. Findings From the European Prospective Investigation Into Cancer and Nutrition–Potsdam Study. Arch Intern Med. 2009;169(15):1355-1362.

9. Olberholtzer L, Dimitri C, Greene C. Price premiums hold on as U.S. organic produce market expands. U.S. Department of Agriculture, Outlook Report Number VGS-308-01, May 2005. Available at "http://www.ers.usda.gov/publications/vgs/may05/VGS30801/" (Accessed on April 25, 2007.)

10. Bosetti C, Spertini L, Parpinel M, Gnagnarella P, Lagiou P, Negri E, et al.Flavonoids and breast cancer risk in Italy. Cancer Epidemiol Biomarkers Prev. 2005;14(4).

11. "http://www.fruitsandveggiesmorematters.org" Accessed June 9, 2010.

12. Anderson SE, Whitaker RC. Prevalence of obesity among US preschool children in different racial and ethnic groups. Arch Pediatr Adolesc Med. 2009 Apr;163(4):344-8.

13. Centers for Disease Control and Prevention, "http://www.cdc.gov" Accessed June 17, 2010.

14. Bouchard MF, Bellinger DC, Wright RO, Weisskopf MG. Attention-Deficit/Hyperactivity Disorder and Urinary Metabolites of Organophosphate Pesticides. Pediatrics.2010;125:e1270–e1277.

15. Dangour AD, Lock K, Havter A, Aikenhead A, Allen E, Uauy R. Nutrition-related health effects of organic foods: a systematic review. Am J Clin Nutr 2010 May 12.

16. "http://www.CalorieKing.com" search accessed 6/9/10 comparing Coca-Cola, Tropicana Orange Juice, Fresh squeezed orange juice, Langer's Blueberry Pomagranate Juice

17. Fiorito LM, Marini M, Francis LA, Smiciklas-Wright H, Birch LL. Beverage intake of girls at age 5 y predicts adiposity and weight status in childhood and adolescence. *Am J Clin Nutr.* 2009 Oct;90(4):935-42.
18. Sak E, Glaser L. Tracking wholesale prices for organic produce. U.S. Department of Agriculture, Economic Research Service. Agricultural Outlook 2001. Available at: HYPERLINK "http://www.ers.usda.gov/publications/agoutlook/oct2001/ao285d.pdf" (Accessed by Up to Date on January 30, 2007).
19. Centers for Disease Control and Prevention. National diabetes fact sheet: general information and national estimates on diabetes in the United States, 2007. Atlanta, GA: U.S. Department of Health and Human Services, Centers for Disease Control and Prevention, 2008.
20. AICR Accessed June 29, 2010 (The New American Plate) www.aicr.org